deconstructing evidence-based practice

This is not a book

the map is not the territory,
the signifier is not the signified...

What deconstruction is not? everything of course!
What is deconstruction? nothing of course!
Jacques Derrida 1983

I know that I have said nothing and will ever say
nothing. And the words don't give a fuck
Jean Genet 1952

I have nothing to say and I am saying it
John Cage 1949

ore rigorous our
ill be the theory that

ame ti
e by saying the
th both voices,
the knock, an
ry carefully
for you to
leas

everything and nothing

deconstructing evidence — based practice

pharmakon,''
, etc? By definition, the list can ne
and I have cited only names, which is inadequate an
for reasons of economy. In fact, I should have cited the
and the interlinking of sentences which in their turn
these names in some of my texts.

What deconstruction is not? everything of course!
What is deconstruction? nothing of course!
I do not think, for all these reasons, that it is a *good wo*
It is certainly not elegant *[beau]*. It has definitely

a book

dawn freshwater

gary rolfe

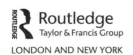

Routledge
Taylor & Francis Group

LONDON AND NEW YORK

First published 2004
by Routledge
2 Park Square, Milton Park, Abingdon, Oxon OX14 4RN

Simultaneously published in the USA and Canada
by Routledge
270 Madison Avenue, New York, NY 10016

Routledge is an imprint of the Taylor & Francis Group

Typeset in Arial, Avant Garde, Courier New and Souvenir by Gary Rolfe
Printed by TJ International, Padstow, UK

British Library Cataloguing in Publication Data
A catalogue record for this book is available from the British Library

Library of Congress Cataloging in Publication Data
A catalog record for this book has been requested

ISBN 0-415-336724 (hardback)
ISBN 0-415-336732 (paperback)

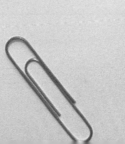

Preface 1
The authority of the 'is'

3

Preface 2
The first time I saw Jacques Derrida

15

Preface 3
The event of a narrative

25

Deconstruction 1
Listen/read/write: an exercise in deconstruction

53

Deconstruction 2
That dangerous supplement ...

87

Deconstruction 3
Analyse this

126

Afterword 1
Rules for reading

153

Afterword 2
Writing in the margins

177

Afterword 3
A tissue of truths

189

Index 217

For Lyn

I repeat, my love: *for you*. I write for you and speak
only to you
Jacques Derrida 1980

Preface

'Here is what I wrote, then read, and what
I am writing that you are going to read.
After which you will again be able to take
possession of this preface which in sum
you have not yet begun to read, even
though, once having read it, you will
already have anticipated everything that
follows and thus you might just as well
dispense with reading the rest.'
(Jacques Derrida   Outwork, prefacing)

Preface 1

The authority of the 'is'

*... perhaps deconstruction would consist, if at least it did consist, in...
deconstructing, dislocating, displacing, disarticulating, disjointing, putting
"out of joint" the authority of the "is".*[1]

---

cont. from p.213/ it pretends to'[2]. All endings, all beginnings, are arbitrary; no, artificial. Let's pretend to begin then.

Before the text
Our explicit intention here has been to write an academic book. That is
not to say, a book that is divorced from practice; on the contrary, we
have tried to write a book that will encourage you to think deeply about
practice and perhaps to change the way you practice as a result of those
thoughts. We appreciate that, to a certain extent, our intention flies in the
face of some current trends, particularly the trend for books and journals
that claim to help the 'busy practitioner' to practice more effectively without having to take the time to do too much reading or thinking.

We do, of course, recognise that many practitioners *are* extremely
busy people who are perhaps so immersed in their day-to-day practice
that they have little time to think, let alone to read. However, we also
believe that to practice is not merely a case of doing, even if it is
'evidence-based doing'. We believe that practice entails reading about
doing, thinking about doing, writing about doing, reading about thinking
about doing, writing about reading about thinking about doing, and
indeed, most other permutations on the above. And until healthcare
workers and their managers recognise, accept and facilitate this expan-

ded concept of practice, they will find it difficult to make the leap from workers to practitioners and from a job to a profession.

We believe that any concept of practice *must* include a reflexive critique of that practice. But herein lies the dilemma, since any practice that looks inwards at itself will only ever be able to judge itself according to its own preestablished criteria. All professions, all disciplines, all discourses include an essence, a set of 'givens' that are seen as being so fundamental that they do not need to be questioned; propositions and beliefs that, as the American constitution says, 'we take to be self-evidently true'. For example, the aim of nursing *is* to care for the sick, the aim of medicine *is* to preserve life, the aim of research *is* to generate knowledge, good practice *is* based on best evidence, and so on. These self-evident first principles are rarely challenged, and represent what the French philosopher Jacques Derrida referred to as 'the authority of the "is"'[3].

Our aim in writing this book is to challenge the authority of the 'is', to initiate a critique of health and social care practice and theory that does not emanate from (and is therefore not bound by the rules of) the practice and theory that it seeks to criticize. For example, we believe that it is important to be able to explore issues of validity and reliability in research without accepting as self-evident that research *is* concerned with the pursuit of knowledge and/or truth. We want to be able to explore ideas of caring in nursing without accepting as self-evident that caring *is* a necessary component of nursing. We want to be able to explore the aims of healthcare without accepting as self-evident that health *is* necessarily a desirable aim in itself. But we also wish to apply this criterion to the very act of criticism itself. We want to explore an approach to critique that is not bound up with the usual rules and expectations of academic scholarship. We believe that what Derrida referred to as 'deconstruction' offers just such an opportunity to step outside of these preconceptions. In an age where evidence-based practice is fast becoming the gold standard in all areas of health and social care, deconstruction highlights the importance of challenging the underlying contradictions that are inherent in *all* texts that contain the evidence which guides our practice. But it goes further: it not only challenges the accepted view of evidence-based practice as the gold standard, it also challenges the *very idea* of a gold standard, of a preferred or authorised way of doing things.

Into the text

In the introduction to his influential book on the theory and practice of
deconstruction, Christopher Norris writes that 'Deconstruction is the
active antithesis of everything that criticism ought to be if one accepts its
traditional values and concepts'[4]. Foremost in the list of traditional values
and concepts is the idea that a text is a representation of a single and (as
far as possible) unambiguous meaning, and that the meaning placed in
the text by its author can be uncovered, elucidated and challenged by
the critic. Deconstruction, then, is the *active* antithesis of this concept. It
seeks not only *intellectually* to undermine the idea of a single fixed
meaning that can be teased out and explored, but also *actively* to
demonstrate the absurdity of that idea by revealing the hidden contradictions and *aporias*[5] inherent in *all* texts, along with the ways in which
authors consciously or unconsciously attempt to conceal those contradictions beneath a seemingly logical and rational façade. Much of the
activity of deconstruction therefore takes place in the 'margins of the
text', in the seemingly innocuous and even superfluous passages where
the author's guard is down. As Norris tells us, 'To "deconstruct" a piece
of writing is therefore to operate a kind of strategic reversal, seizing on
precisely those unregarded details (casual metaphors, footnotes, inciden-
tal turns of argument) which are always and necessarily, passed over by
interpreters of a more orthodox persuasion'[6].

Deconstruction is a response not only to the idea of an authoritarian
text (that is, a text that upholds the authority of the 'is', a text which
claims to 'tell it like it *is*'), but also to the idea of an authoritative
approach to critiquing that text, and in particular, to the doctrine of
structuralism, which seeks to provide a more or less scientific method for
what was previously regarded as the *art* of criticism. The structuralists, as
upholders of the traditional values of criticism, advocate a single method
in order to uncover a single meaning in the text. In contrast, deconstruction shuns the idea of a single method. As Roland Barthes, a structuralist-
turned-post-structuralist, observed: 'At a *certain moment,* therefore, it is
necessary to turn against Method, or at least to treat it without any
founding privilege as one of the voices of plurality'[7]. Norris goes even
further to suggest that deconstruction does not seek to replace Method
with multiple methods, but rather to reject the very notion. Deconstruction is therefore less a method and more a perspective. It involves a
certain way of thinking about texts and about itself (what might be called

an interpretive self-consciousness) that troubles the underpinning assumptions of the text. It challenges the notion of wholeness within texts, arguing that all representation is partial. The internal fissures of the text are revealed not only through what is written; fault lines are also detected within the silences, the gaps, the margins, the *aporias* and between the lines.

We can see, then, that 'To present "deconstruction" as if it were a method, a system or a settled body of ideas would be to falsify its nature and lay oneself open to charges of reductive misunderstanding'[8]. This clearly offers a challenge to the would-be deconstructionist: if there is no method, then what exactly is deconstruction and how is it to be learnt and practised? We might turn to Jaques Derrida, the 'founder' of deconstruction, for an answer. However, he tells us merely that 'deconstruction loses nothing from admitting that it is impossible'[9]. In fact the *act* of deconstruction is, in one sense, unnecessary, since a 'deconstructive reading attends to the deconstructive processes *always* occurring in the texts and *already* there waiting to be read'[10]. The deconstructive process comes not from the reader/critic but from the text itself; it is already there, it is the tension 'between what [the text] manifestly *means to say* and what it is nonetheless *constrained to mean*'[11]. To say that deconstruction is impossible is therefore to acknowledge 'the impossible desire of language ... to make present the permanently elusive'[12].

There is no method to deconstruction because texts *literally* deconstruct themselves in their impossible attempt to employ language as a 'transcendental signifier'[13], that is, as a way of 'pointing' at some eternal truth or other. As Spivak observes, 'All texts ... are rehearsing their grammatological structure, self-deconstructing as they constitute themselves'[14]. All that the budding deconstructionist needs to do, then, is write, since in the final analysis, deconstruction *is* writing. Furthermore, it is writing with no preconceived goal; as Roland Barthes put it, '*to write* is an intransitive verb'[15], a verb without an object, an end in itself. Deconstruction manifests itself in the *process* of writing rather than in the product: 'Deconstruction *takes place*, it is an *event* that does not await the deliberation, consciousness, or organization of a subject'[16].

But if this is indeed the case, then deconstruction is impossible in another and more tangible sense. Firstly, of course, the process of deconstructive writing produces a second text as a supplement to that which it seeks to deconstruct, which is itself (in Spivak's words) self-deconstructing as it constitutes itself (what we might call the process of being re-invented whilst simultaneously being invented). Secondly, as we have seen, there is no single authoritative and 'correct' deconstructive reading/writing of any particular text. Therefore, each text contains within itself the possibility of a vast number of supplementary deconstructive texts, and each of those is likewise open to further deconstruction *ad infinitum* in an infinite regress. As Spivak points out, 'The fall into the abyss of deconstruction inspires us with as much pleasure as fear. We are intoxicated with the prospect of never hitting bottom'[17]. But we do not even need to *write* in order to fall into the abyss. The very act of reading creates a new and different text; that is to say, *reading writes*. To deconstruct a text is therefore to embark on an endless (and thus, in a sense, an impossible) journey, in which the destination is constantly revised as soon as it is realised. It is a leap in the dark in the knowledge that you might never again set foot on solid ground, indeed, you might even begin to question if there ever was solid ground.

We can see, then, that although deconstruction is first and foremost a way of writing, it is a particular kind of writing that transgresses many of the accepted rules of 'good' academic scholarship. Unlike most academic writing, deconstruction is not concerned with the clear communication of a single authoritative message. In fact, it seeks to undermine the very notion of the possibility of clear communication, since 'meaning and language undermine each other ... for language is not the vehicle of meaning but its destroyer'[18]. As Derrida asks:

> Is it certain that there corresponds to the word *communication* a unique, univocal concept, a concept that can be rigorously grasped and transmitted: a communicable concept? Following a strange figure of discourse, one must first ask whether the word or signifier 'communication' communicates a determined content, an identifiable meaning, a describable value.[19]

Deconstruction, then, is the enemy of clear and straightforward communication; it seeks out the parts of the text where communication *inevitably* breaks down. But not only does deconstructive writing undermine the idea of straightforward communication in the texts it seeks to critique; it is itself often obscure and demanding of the reader in ways far beyond the simple transmission and understanding of meaning. Deconstructive writing is concerned with asking rather than answering questions; it attempts to engage the reader in a creative partnership; it is catalytic rather than communicative, and seeks to empower rather than instruct. As Barthes observed, the author (that is, the singular, authoritative voice that 'tells it like it is') is dead[20], and the aim of deconstructive writing is to transform the reader into her own author, into a deconstructive *rewriter*. As we have seen, *reading writes*.

But deconstructive writing not only transgresses the boundaries of content; it also often steps outside of the accepted notions of form; indeed, the *very idea* of the book is pushed to its limits. As Derrida points out, in questioning (deconstructing) the function of writing, we must also question (deconstruct) the function of the presentation of writing, and since writing is *reflexive*, the writing that questions the form and function of writing must itself step outside of the form and function that it is questioning. In other words, it is not possible to write a traditional book that questions the form and function of the traditional book: 'the book form alone can no longer settle ... the case of those writing processes which, in *practically* questioning that form, must also dismantle it'[21]. Deconstruction puts its money where its mouth is; it practices what it preaches; in *practically* questioning the form and content of writing and of the book, it also dismantles it.

Beyond the text

We have seen that the purpose of deconstruction is not the simple, clear communication of ideas from writer to reader; rather, the purpose of deconstruction is dissemination, change, action, reflection, and to challenge the 'self-evident' beliefs and assumptions of academic scholarship. This can be an uncomfortable process, not least because we are confronted with ourselves and our practices; deconstruction knows our hiding places and remorselessly exposes them.

Deconstruction is therefore not only concerned with texts. Or rather, deconstruction aims to stretch the idea of the text beyond its natural limits to include *all* attempts at representation. By unsettling the 'givens' with which we have surrounded ourselves, not only is our account of the world challenged, but also our account of ourselves. In other words, deconstruction involves the dissolution of the self as a single stable image, it *precedes* the process of construction(ism) in which the many 'selves' that we have always been are permitted to become. Self is therefore deconstructed and reconstructed through the process of writing and reading texts, and deconstruction offers an opportunity to engage in reflexive dialogue with self and others. Self as an authority is challenged whilst simultaneously becoming an authority; self is inventing itself through writing whilst being invented by the text. As Roland Barthes so succinctly put it: 'I am writing a text and I call it R.B.'[22].

The self, then, is constantly in creation and co-creation with others and with the environment, and this co-creation leads to the acknowledgement of multiple selves which are always becoming and never ending. Like written texts, the notion of the solid ground of the self is contested, thereby allowing, indeed, impelling, the writer to be written by her[23] writing, and the practitioner to be transformed by her caring interventions by and with her patients. In this sense, deconstruction is not unlike psychoanalysis. As Sarap[24] points out, the 'close reading' of a text is 'very similar to psychoanalytic approaches to neurotic symptoms', whilst Norris contends that Derrida 'is proposing what amounts to a psychoanalysis of Western "logocentric" reason'[25]. It is certainly true that Derrida initiated an intense interest amongst deconstructionists in the work of Freud and other psychotherapists, and this interest has more recently been reciprocated by a number of psychotherapists who have started to look at (verbal and non-verbal) conversations as texts to be deconstructed[26].

If psychoanalysis works as a psychological metaphor for deconstruction, then a commonly used physical metaphor is that of the X-ray. Derrida sees written texts as (metaphorically) composed of layers of references and citations, as 'an infinite number of booklets enclosing and fitting inside other booklets, which are only able to issue forth by grafting, sampling, quotations, epigraphs, references, etc'[27], one written over the top of the other, each acknowledging the influence of the one immediately below it, whilst at the same time acting to obscure it. The deconstructive reading of a text is thus likened to an X-ray photograph which discovers or makes visible the layers of textual references which were previously hidden below the surface.

> Reading then resembles those X-Ray pictures which discover, under the epidermis of the last painting, another hidden picture: the same painter or another painter, no matter, who would himself, for want of materials, or for a new effect, use the substance of an ancient canvas

or conserve the fragment of a first sketch. And beneath *that*, etc...[28]

Other metaphors employ such images as space: Fox[29], for example, likens deconstruction to the shift from striated space (which has hiding places) to smooth space in which horizons and edges come into view. What all these metaphors have in common is that they describe a bringing of something that was previously (wittingly or unwittingly) concealed into the foreground. Hence subtext is turned into text and texts within text are made explicit. Further, to deconstruct locates 'culture', with all its hidden agendas, biases and inequalities, chaos and disorder, conflict and secrets, at the centre of a text.

Subverting the text
Deconstruction therefore looks beyond the traditional notion of the written text. Whilst it aims to identify the author, her influence and her contradictions, it also attempts to make explicit the embedded cultural, traditional and contextual dissonance inherent in *all* texts. As previously mentioned, this can and does cause some discomfort (and excitement) for those engaged in the deconstructive endeavour. If tradition is the illusion of permanence, then deconstruction troubles us to let go of the illusion, to settle for being unsettled, to agree to be consistently inconsistent and to be open to transformation. Giddens[30] comments that through deconstruction, tradition loses its force and agency, and, transformed by reflexivity, becomes emancipated.

Herein lies another paradox for the deconstructionist to battle with, for whilst deconstruction aims to examine the hidden hierarchies within a text, it also rejects dialectical critique and abandons emancipatory movement[31]. On the one hand it is political, in that it has radical political implications, and yet, just as deconstruction turns away from method, Derrida also views it as a retreat from any kind of direct confrontational politics[32]. It is political precisely because it is apolitical; it refuses to play by the traditional rules of the game of politics, recognising that those rules stack the odds in favour of those already in power. As Spivak notes: 'Deconstruction cannot found a political program of any kind.... deconstruction suggests that there is no absolute justification of *any* position'[33]. Thus, by refusing to play power games, deconstruction offers the potential for liberation from the inherent social and cultural constructions of power.

Rather than becoming involved in power struggles, deconstruction is concerned with the analysis and exposure of the systems of binary opposites that prop up the hierarchy and which are inherent (and often disguised) in all texts. Derrida argues that these binary pairs are always presented in such a way that one of the terms is seen as superior to the other, for example 'Theory:practice', 'Doctor:nurse', 'Health:illness', and so on. For Derrida, the *primary* binary pair, from which all others spring, is 'Speech:writing', and he devoted much of his early work to exploring the unchallenged primacy of the spoken word over the written word (what he called logocentrism) in some of the key texts of Western philosophy. However, rather than simply inverting the binary pair, Derrida attempted to show how each is dependent on and contained within the other, so that neither is possible without its seeming opposite. The power structure that the text is attempting to promote is therefore subverted by demonstrating how the seeds of the argument against the power structure are concealed just below the surface.

A note on the author(ity) of the text

If Barthes is right and the author is dead, then who is writing this text? On the face of it (that is, on the cover of the book), it has two writers; two authors. But that, of course, is only half the story: for the deconstructionists, all texts are intertexts; all texts take their meaning only in relation to other texts; more than that, all texts *are* all other texts, are nothing but a series of (literal and figurative) *quotations* from other texts; 'the text is a tissue of quotations drawn from the innumerable centres of culture.... the writer can only imitate a gesture that is always anterior, never original. His only power is to mix writings, to counter the ones with the others, in such a way as never to rest on any of them'[34]. Do you see?

So, on one level, this text has two authors but innumerable writers. But on another level, the *book* might well have two authors, but the *text* can only ever have one. The text you are reading now was *not* written by two authors consecutively pressing the keys of the word processor; it has a *single* author (I won't tell you which). Similarly for the entire text that comprises this book: every word, most paragraphs and some entire chapters were the work of a single author. And even where collaboration took place, it fell to one or other of us to transcribe (and inevitably to add to) that collaborative text.

It therefore feels somewhat dishonest to continue to write in the plural, to refer to myself as 'we'. The rest of this book is therefore written

in the first person: *I* address *you* directly. You might, if you wish, attempt
to discover the 'I' that is writing any particular sentence; there are certainly some clues in the text; but it is not that important, and I suspect that
you are not particularly interested. In any case, this is an intertext which
probably contains more original ideas from Derrida than from Freshwater
or Rolfe.

Notes

1   Derrida, J. The time is out of joint. In A. Haverkamp (ed) *Decon-
    struction is/in America: A New Sense of the Political*, New York: New
    York University Press, 1995, p.25
2   Derrida, J. Living on: border lines. In H. Bloom et al. (eds)
    Deconstruction and Criticism, London: Routledge & Kegan Paul,
    1979, pp.96-7
3   Ibid., p.25
4   Norris, C. *Deconstruction Theory and Practice (revised edition)*,
    London: Routledge, 1991, p.xi
5   Norris (ibid., p.49) tells us that *'Aporia* derives from the Greek word
    meaning "unpassable path".... What deconstruction persistently
    reveals is an ultimate impasse of thought engendered by a rhetoric
    that always insinuates its own textual workings into the truth claims
    of philosophy'.
6   Norris, C. *Derrida*, London: Fontana, 1987, p.19
7   Barthes, R. Writers, intellectuals, teachers. In R. Barthes *Image Music
    Text*, London: Fontana, 1977, p.201, italics in original
8   Norris 1991, op. cit., p.1
9   Derrida, J. (1987) Psyche: inventions of the other. In P. Kamuf (ed)
    A Derrida Reader: Reading Between the Blinds, New York:
    Harvester Wheatsheaf, 1991, p. 209
10 Payne, M. *Reading Theory*, Oxford: Blackwell, 1993, p.121, italics in
    original
11 Norris 1987, op. cit., p.19, italics in original
12 Payne, op. cit., p.121
13 Usher, R. & Edwards, R. *Postmodernism and Education*, London:
    Routledge, 1994, p.144

14 Spivak, G.C. Translator's preface. In Derrida, J. *Of Grammatology*, Baltimore: The Johns Hopkins University Press, 1976, p.lxxviii

15 Barthes, R. To write: an intransitive verb. In R. Macksey & E. Donato (eds) *The Language of Criticism and the Sciences of Man*, Baltimore: Johns Hopkins University Press, 1970

16 Derrida, J. (1983) Letter to a Japanese Friend. In P. Kamuf, *A Derrida Reader*, New York: Harvester, 1991, p.274, my italics

17 Spivak, op. cit., p.lxxvii

18 Delanty, G. *Modernity and Postmodernity*. London: Sage, 2000, p.140

19 Derrida, J. (1971) Signature Event Context. In J. Derrida, *Margins of Philosophy*, New York: Harvester Wheatsheaf, 1982, p.309

20 Barthes, R. (1968) The death of the author. In R. Barthes *Image Music Text*, London: Fontana, 1977

21 Derrida, J. (1972) *Dissemination*, London: Athlone, 1981, p.3

22 Barthes, R. (1975) *Roland Barthes*, Basingstoke: Macmillan, 1995, p.56

23 As we shall see (page 11), one of the functions of deconstruction is to dismantle 'binary pairs' of the type He:she. However, in some cases, especially where a power dynamic is involved, Derrida argues that binary pairs must be reversed before they can be overturned (see page 161). Our fear, then, is that if we attempt to write in gender-neutral language,, the male polarity will simply reassert itself by stealth back into the text, if not by the writer, then by the reader. For this reason, we intend to use female gendered pronouns throughout this book.

24 Sarap, M. *An Introductory Guide to Post Structuralism and Postmodernism*, Hemel Hempstead: Harvester, 1993, p.50

25 Norris, C. (1989) Deconstruction, post-modernism and the visual arts. In M. McQuillan (ed) *Deconstruction: A Reader*, Edinburgh: Edinburgh University Press, 2000, p.109

26 Chaplin, J. *The Rhythm Model*. In I. Bruna Seu and M. Colleen Heenan (eds) *Feminism and Psychotherapy*, London: Sage, 1998, Chapter 8

27 Derrida, J. The double session. In J. Derrida *Dissemination*, op. cit., p.223

28 Derrida, J. *Dissemination*, op. cit., p.357

29 Fox, N. J. *Beyond Health: Postmodernism and Embodiment*, London: Free Association Books, 1999

30 Giddens, A. Modernity and self identity: self and society in the late modern age. In F. Frascina & J. Harris (eds) *Art in Modern Culture*, London: Phaidon Press, 1994

31 Derrida, J. Forces of law: the mystical foundation of authority. In D. Cornell, M. Rosenfeld & D.G. Carlson (eds) *Deconstruction and the Possibility of Justice*, New York: Routledge, 1992

32 Ibid.

33 Spivak, G. Practical politics of the open end, *Canadian Journal of Political and Social Theory*, 12, 1-2, pp.104-11, 1988, p.104

34 Barthes (1968) The death of the author, op. cit., p.146

Preface 2

The first time I saw Jacques Derrida

This interweaving, this textile, is the text produced only in the transformation of another text[1].

Deconstruction, as you have seen, is a way of writing; not a *particular* way of writing, but nevertheless a way that is different from the standard academic format. Deconstruction has its own style(s), its own structure(s), its own form(s). It challenges not only the *content* of the text, not only the *style* in which the text is written, but the very *form* that it takes. Deconstruction (you will recall) challenges the very idea of the book; deconstructive texts deconstruct themselves.

I might therefore begin by deconstructing the idea of a preface. I could point out, for example, that the preface occupies a curious 'third place', neither part of, nor separate from, the book, 'neither in the markings, nor in the marchings, nor in the margins, of the book'[2]. If deconstruction consists in uncovering the contradictions hidden in all texts, then I could discuss how all prefaces are built upon a lie, that the *prae-fatio*, the 'saying before-hand', is always written retrospectively, and that 'the preface would announce in the future tense ('this is what you are going to read') the conceptual content or significance ... of what will *already* have been *written*'[3], or simply 'Here is what I wrote, then read, and what I am writing that you are going to read'[4].

I could further show that the idea of the preface is the mirror of the idea of deconstruction, that 'A preface would retrace and presage here a *general* theory and practice of deconstruction'[5], that the preface is *itself* a deconstruction, and that 'each reading of the "text" is a preface to the next'[6].

I could continue by citing the opening sentence of Derrida's own preface to *Dissemination*: 'This (therefore) will not have been a book'[7], and show how this single sentence contains the seed (semen) of the entire book: 'as presentation ("this"), anticipation ("will"), negation ("not"), recapitulation ("have been"), and conclusion ("therefore")'[8].

But of course that has already been done, so I will begin instead with someone else's preface, or rather, with the writing of someone else *as* a preface. The French/Algerian writer and philosopher Hélène Cixous describes her first encounter with the work of Jacques Derrida:

> The first time I saw Jacques Derrida (it must have been in 1962) he was walking fast and sure along a mountain's crest, from left to right, I was at Arachon, I was reading (it must have been *Force et significa-tion*), from where I was I could see him clearly advancing black on the clear sky, feet on a tightrope, the crest was terribly sharp, he was walking along the peak, from far away I saw it, his hike along the line between mountain and sky which were melting into each other, he had to travel a path no wider than a pencil stroke.
>
> He wasn't running, fast, he was *making* his way, *all* the way along the crests. Going from left to right, according to the (incarnate) pace of writing. Landscape without any border other than, at each instant, displacing him from his pace. Before him, nothing but the great stand-ing air. I had never seen someone from our century write like this, on the world's cutting edge, the air had the air of a transparent door, so entirely open one had to search for the stiles ...[9]

The first time *I* saw Jacques Derrida... No, let me rephrase that. The first JD that I saw (it must have been 1996) was digging, burrowing, not so much from left to right as downwards, deep into the heart of some-thing. Not digging himself deeper into a hole, but digging a hole for others (and himself) to fall into: *une abîme*, as he would call it; an abyss. I was reading *Of Grammatology* at the time, at the behest of Max van Manen. Van Manen[10] had taught me about writing, and in particular, how writing is a means as well as an end. He encouraged me to explore the process of writing and the ways in which it differs from speech. He introduced me first to Roland Barthes and then to Jacques Derrida.

The first time I saw Barthes, he was ambling, meandering, strolling, taking in the scenery, whereas, as I said, Derrida was burrowing. Barthes was writing *himself* when I first saw him ('I am writing a text, and I call it RB'[11], as he famously said); Derrida was just writing. That is to say, he was writing a text. But that is also to say that he was doing far more than *writing* a *text*, if by writing we mean 'to make letters or other symbols on a surface, especially with a pen or pencil on paper', or even 'to compose in written form for publication', and if by a text we mean 'the wording of something written or printed' or 'the main body of a book or page'[12]. No, the first JD that I saw was doing far more than that. He had to be, since, as he himself pointed out, *'il n'y a pas de hors-texte'*[13]. In a sense, then, all of life is an act of writing. But this is (probably) not quite what JD meant. He was not trying to claim (as some would have it) that 'there is nothing outside the text', that the world is nothing but text; rather, he was suggesting that 'there is no outside-text', that once you fall into the abyss of (a) text, there are no external reference points, only references to other texts. Thus:

> reading ... cannot legitimately transgress the text toward something other than it, toward a referent (a reality that is metaphysical, histor-ical, psychobiographical, etc.) or toward a signified outside the text whose content could take place, could have taken place outside of language, that is to say, in the sense that we give here to the word, outside of writing in general[14].

Texts (as you already know) can be understood only in relation to other texts, as interwoven threads, as textile.

But if texts function *in relation* to each other, then they function differently in different situations. A text might, on one occasion, act as a con-text, as a (more or less failed) attempt to fix meaning, to signify something outside itself; on another occasion as a pre-text, an introduc-tion or leading-in to some other text; and on another occasion as a sub-text, a burrowing below the surface of the text. It is all a matter of per-spective. Sometimes these functions become blurred, sometimes they shift. One of the texts in this book was originally published in a journal as sub-text, as a deconstruction of some other texts. Here, it functions as con-text, as the source of a further sub-text; as you have seen, 'each reading of the "text" is a preface to the next'.

To make life easier for you, the texts in this book are coded by the use of different typefaces. This is a strategy that Derrida is also fond of (*see*, for example, *Dissemination*[15] and *Glas*[16]), although he rarely provides a key to his typographics. The key employed in this book is simple. Most chapters in this book begin with a pre-text, a leading-in, which is also a pretext, an excuse (but also a concealment) for what follows. The text you are now reading is a pre-text, and is denoted by this standard serif typeface. All chapters include a con-text, a thesis, which also provides the context, situation or 'original meaning' of the chapter. The con-text is denoted by this sanserif typeface. However, you have seen that Derrida (along with Barthes) rejects the idea of original authorial meaning in favour of a multiplicity of meanings that are 'read in' by the multiple readers of the text. Most of the chapters therefore also include at least one sub-text, a deconstructive excavation of the con-text, a burrowing into its subconscious, which is also a subtext, an occult or hidden mean-ing, one of many (an infinitude?) alternative readings. `The sub-text is denoted by this typewriter-like font to remind you that deconstruction is first and foremost an act of writ-ing`. In addition to the micro level of the individual chapters, the book as a whole is also divided into three parts that function as pre-text, con-text and sub-text on a macro level. Pre-text: before the text, explaining deconstruction, justifying it, providing it with a pretext. Con-text: with the text, *weaving together* deconstruction and evidence-based practice, situating it, providing it with a context. `Sub-text: beneath the text, delving into the foundations of deconstruction, exploring its roots, providing it with a subtext.`

| | | **EVIDENCE-BASED PRACTICE** | | |
		reading	*writing*	**practising**
D E C O N S T R U C T I O N	pre-text	The authority of the 'is'	*The first time I saw Jacques Derrida*	**The event of a narrative**
	con-text	Listen/read/write: an exercise in deconstruction	*That dangerous supplement...*	Analyse this
	sub-text	`Rules for reading`	`Writing in the margins`	`A tissue of truths`

A matrix; that is to say, *une matrice*, a womb[17]; that is to say, an arrangement, a structure for giving birth to a text, to a series of texts, to a child: 'writings: those stillborn children one sends oneself in order to stop hearing about them - precisely because children are first of all what one wishes to hear speak by themselves'[18]. *Un enfant*: from the Latin *infans*, meaning 'unable to talk', to remind us that writing does not speak, that writing is not speech.

A matrix, then; that is to say, rows and columns, warp and weft, woven together; that is to say, a tissue[19], a textile, a text[20], weaving the weft of deconstruction with the warp of evidence-based practice. A textile of writing and practice: 'The *interweaving* of language, the interweaving of that which is purely language in language with the other threads of experience constitutes a cloth'[21]. This book, this collection of texts, is presented horizontally, along the warp (along the axis of *deconstruction*); that is, as pre-text(s) followed by con-text(s) followed by sub-text(s). On the face of it, a book about deconstruction, but shot through with the weft of evidence-based practice; that is, of reading, followed by *writing*, followed by **practising**.

As well as this typographic strategy, I borrow another textual device from Derrida, and that is his predilection for presenting parallel texts in separate columns on the same page. His first use of this device was in the essay 'The double session', originally published in 1970 in the literary journal *Tel Quel*[22], and later as part of his book *Dissemination*[23], in which passages from Plato and Mallarmé are presented side-by-side on a single page. He used the double column again, more extensively, in an essay entitled 'Tympan', originally published in 1972 in his book *The Margins of Philosophy*[24]. As you have already seen, one of the recurring themes in Derrida's work is his obsession with what he calls 'the margins of the text', in the sense both of the parts of the text that other critics overlook, the footnotes, the jokey asides; and also of the way that one of the terms in a pair of binary opposites is often marginalised in favour of the other. In 'Tympans', the theme of margins is employed both metaphorically and literally in what becomes a spiral labyrinth.

Metaphorically, 'Tympans' is an investigation into the marginalisation of the term 'outer' of the binary pair 'inner:outer'. In the left hand column is the philosophical discussion of the inner and the outer that begins: 'To tympanize - philosophy', with a translators note pointing out that 'In French, *tympaniser* is an archaic verb meaning to criticize, to ridicule publicly'[25]. In the right hand column is a long quotation from the memoirs of the writer Michel Leiris which meditates on the spiral shape in nature. This juxtaposition of two seemingly unrelated texts points to another theme running throughout the work of Derrida, that of the play on similar sounding words. In this case, the play is clearly on the word *tympaniser*, to critique, and also the tympanic membrane, which encloses the *spiral shaped* cochlea of the *inner* ear. You might also note that the quotation from Leiris is from a chapter entitled 'Persephone' and that one of its subjects is the earwig, the *perce-oreille* (literally, ear-piercer), which not only *sounds* similar to *Persephone*, but also continues the theme of the outer and the inner, and in particular, of the attempts to reinstate the marginalised term (outer) as equal to its binary opposite (inner) (that is, of the attempt of the outer to pierce the inner). You can see, then, that Derrida intends his writing to operate on many different metaphoric levels.

Tympan

other on either side of the membrane? How to block this correspondence destined to weaken, muffle, forbid the blows from the outside, the other hammer? The "hammer that speaks" to him "who has the third ear" (*der das dritte Ohr hat*). How to interpret—but here interpretation can no longer be a theory or discursive practice of philosophy—the strange and unique property of a discourse that organizes the *economy* of its representation, the law of its proper weave, such that *its* outside is never its *outside*, never surprises it, such that the logic of its heteronomy still reasons from within the vault of its autism?

For this is how *Being* is understood: its proper. It assures without let-up the *relevant* movement of reappropriation. Can one then pass this singular limit which is not a limit, which no more separates the inside from the outside than it assures their permeable and transparent continuity? What form could this play of limit/passage have, this logos which posits and negates itself in permitting its own voice to well up? Is this a well-put question?

The analyses that give rise to one another in this book do not answer this question, bringing to it neither an answer nor *an* answer. They work, rather, to transform and displace its statement, and toward examining the presuppositions of the question, the institution of its protocol, the laws of its procedure, the headings of its alleged homogeneity, of its apparent unicity; can one treat of philosophy itself (metaphysics itself, that is, ontotheology) without already permitting the dictation, along with the pretention to unity and unicity, of the ungraspable and imperial totality of an order? If there are margins, is there still a philosophy, *the* philosophy?

No answer, then. Perhaps, in the long run, not even a question. The copulative correspondence, the opposition question/answer is already lodged

xvi

which occasionally, so they say, perforates human tympanums with its pincers, has in common with the daughter of Demeter that it too buries itself in a subterranean kingdom. The deep country of hearing, described in terms of geology more than in those of any other natural science, not only by virtue of the cartilaginous cavern that constitutes its organ, but also by virtue of the relationship that unites it to grottoes, to chasms, to all the pockets hollowed out of the terrestrial crust whose emptiness makes them into resonating drums for the slightest sounds. Just as one might worry about the idea of the tympanum, a fragile *membrane* threatened with perforations by the minute pincers of an insect—unless it had

But as I have said, the theme of the margin is also played out literally, since the text is arranged on the page as two unequal columns, one of which appears to be the margin of the other. As Peggy Kamuf points out:

> By means of these typographics, Derrida contrives to proliferate the margins on which and in which he is writing. In its much narrower column, the Leiris quotation appears to be written in the margin of Derrida's column on the left, whereas the space between the two is a thin blank column running down the right third

of the page[26].

She continues:

> Although Derrida never explicitly refers to the quotation, it incessantly crosses over the minimal barrier set up to its left and intrudes on the space reserved for the introductory discourse[27].

What, then, is the relationship between these texts? Is Derrida's writing a pre-text to Leiris or is it a deconstructive sub-text? Or, indeed, is there some other relationship? As I have said, Derrida gives very few clues.

I turn now to Derrida's other and more famous/notorious deployment of parallel texts in columns on the same page. *Glas*[28], first published in French in 1974 and translated into English 12 years later, is a far more ambitious project. For one thing, it is an entire book, and for another, there are at least three different typefaces employed in it. As Kamuf observes:

> One way to describe *Glas* is simply to invoke its volume: 100 cubic inches (10 x 10 x 1 in the original edition). On its large, squared pages, two wide columns face off in different type: smaller, denser on the left, larger, more spaced out on the right. Thumb through the pages and you will see a third type, the smallest of the three, cutting

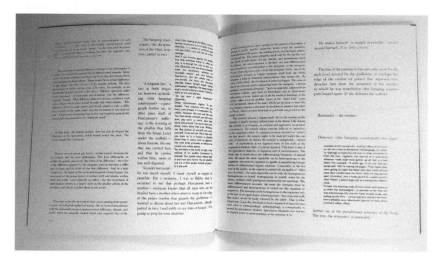

into the column at various points, forming inscribed incisions either along its outermost edge, or down the center. There are no notes, no chapter headings, no table of contents. Each column begins in what appears to be the middle of a sentence and ends, 283 pages further on, without any final punctuation[29].

Or, as Derrida puts it, in the right-hand column of page 1 (the square brackets contain translators' notes):

> Two unequal columns, they say distyle [disent-ils], each of which - envelop(e)(s) or sheath(es), incalculably reverses, turns inside out, replaces, remarks, overlaps [recoupe] the other[30].

And as Kamuf continues, 'What is going on here? Clearly many things at once, too many ever to allow anything but a very partial description'[31]. Many critics of Derrida simply do not 'get' what is going on, and dismiss his work as a triumph of style over content. However, for Derrida, content, style and form cannot be separated; what is written, the stylistic form that the writing takes, and the physical presentation of the writing are all of equal importance. I shall explore this theme in more detail in *Preface 3* and again in *Afterword 2*, but let us now briefly turn to a rather more straightforward use of alternative presentations of text. Derrida was not the first writer to organize his text in parallel columns. Two decades before 'Tympan', the American novelist John Barth, in Chapter 20 of his novel *The Floating Opera*, wrote:

> My prose is a plodding, graceless thing, and I've no comprehension of stylistic tricks. Nevertheless I must begin this chapter in two voices, because it requires two separate introductions delivered simultaneously.

It's not so difficult, is it, to read two columns at the same time? I'll commence by saying the same thing with both voices, so, until you've got the knack, and then separate them ever so gradually until you're used to	It's not so difficult, is it, to read two columns at the same time? I'll commence by saying the same thing with both voices, so, until you've got the knack, and then part them very carefully until it's no trouble for you to

keeping two distinct narrative voices in your head at the same time.

Ready? Well: when I re-entered my office the clock in the tower of the Municipal Building was just striking two...

follow both sets of ideas simultaneously and accurately.

Ready? Well: you'll recall that chapter before last I declared to Mister Haecker that anyone who wishes...[32]

Have you got the knack? In *Preface 3* you will have the opportunity to put your new-found reading skills to the test.

Notes

1   Derrida, J. (1972) *Positions*, Chicago: University of Chicago Press, 1982
2   Derrida, J. (1972) *Dissemination*, London: Athlone, 1981, p.15
3   Ibid., p.7, emphasis in original
4   Ibid., p.7
5   Ibid., p.7
6   Spivak, G.C. Translator's preface. In J. Derrida (1967) *Of Grammatology*, Baltimore: The Johns Hopkins University Press, 1976, p.xll
7   Derrida (1972) *Dissemination*, op. cit., p.3
8   Johnson, B. Translator's preface. In Derrida, ibid., p.xxxii
9   Cixous, H. (1994) What is it o'clock? Or the door (we never enter). In H. Cixous *Stigmata*, London: Routledge, 1998, p.57
10 van Manen, M. (1990) *Researching Lived Experience*, Ontario: Althouse, 1997
11 Barthes, R. (1975) *Roland Barthes*, Basingstoke: Macmillan, 1995, p.56
12 *Oxford Paperback Dictionary*, Oxford: OUP
13 Derrida, J. (1967) *Of Grammatology*, op. cit., p.158
14 Ibid., p.158
15 Derrida (1972) *Dissemination*, op. cit.
16 Derrida, J. (1986) *Glas*, Lincoln: University of Nebraska Press, 1990
17 See translator's note in Derrida, J. *Points...*, Stanford: Stanford University Press, 1995, p.90

18 Derrida, J. (1980) *The Postcard: From Socrates to Freud and Beyond*, Chicago: The University of Chicago Press, 1987, p.25

19 Tissue, from the early French *tissu*, woven

20 Text, from the Latin *texere*, to weave

21 Derrida, J. (1967) Form and meaning: a note on the phenomenology of language. In J. Derrida, *Margins of Philosophy*, New York: Harvester Wheatsheaf, 1982, p.160

22 Derrida, J. The double session, *Tel Quel*, whole issues 41 & 42

23 Derrida, J. (1970) The double session. In *Dissemination*, op. cit., pp.173-285

24 Derrida, J. (1972) Tympan. In J. Derrida *Margins of Philosophy*, New York: Harvester Wheatsheaf, 1982, pp.ix-xxix

25 Ibid., p.x

26 Kamuf, P. (ed) *A Derrida Reader: Between the Blinds*, New York: Harvester Wheatsheaf, p.146

27 Ibid., p.146

28 Derrida *Glas*, op. cit.

29 Kamuf, op. cit., p.315

30 Derrida Glas, op. Cit., p.1

31 Kamuf, op. cit., p.315

32 Barth, J. (1956) *The Floating Opera*, New York: Bantam, 1972, p.168

Preface 3

The event of a narrative

What is a narrative - this thing that we call a narrative? Does it take place? Where and when? What might the taking-place or the event of a narrative be?[1]

'This (therefore) will not have been a book', not a conventional book, or at least, not *structured* in a conventional manner. Part of what makes its structure unconventional is that it contains three prefaces; part of the reason for three prefaces is to ease you into the unconventional structure and style of a book with

'While the form of the "book" is now going through a period of general upheaval, and while that form now appears less natural, and its history less transparent, than ever, and while one cannot tamper with it without disturbing everything else, the book form alone can no longer settle - here for example - the case of those writing processes which, in *practically* questioning that form, must also dismantle it.' (Derrida - Dissemination, p.3)

three prefaces. The first two of these prefaces employed a more or less traditional format and style: in the first, I introduced you to some of the thinking behind deconstruction; in the second, I explored some alternative ways of organising and presenting the text. However, as McLuhan told us nearly forty years ago, the medium is the message, although we are rarely aware that it is so. Thus, 'the "content" of a medium is like the juicy piece of meat carried by the burglar to distract the watchdog of the mind'[2]. It is only when our expectations of the medium are deliberately transgressed that we see what is normally invisible to us, that the way in which the message is delivered, its 'subliminal charge'[3], is at least as important as the message itself.

A constant theme throughout Derrida's work has been his insistence that speech and writing are very different media which produce very different effects, but that writing has come to be seen as merely a supplement to speech, as nothing more than a record of the spoken word.

'Now we must think that writing is at the same time more exterior to speech, not being its "image" or its "symbol", and more interior to speech, which is already in itself a writing.' (Derrida - Of Grammatology, p.46)

In this third preface, I aim not only to explore some of these differences between writing and speech (content), but to transgress the usual presentation of written texts (style and form) so that you might be constantly reminded that this is a text and not a transcription of (a) speech. My way of surfacing the 'subliminal charge' of the medium is to borrow Derrida's strategy of presenting two different but related texts in parallel columns. There is a further irony, however, since the left hand column actually *is* a transcription of a speech, albeit a speech (in part) about writing. But there is another reason for the unusual form of this third preface, since, as we saw in *Preface 2*, for Derrida it is not only the *presentation*, but the very *idea* of a preface that is problematic. As Alan Bass, one of Derrida's translators, reminds us:

'When a text quotes and requotes, with or without quotation marks, when it is written on the brink, you start, or indeed have already started, to lose your footing. You lose sight of any demarcation between a text and what is outside it.' (Derrida - Living on: border lines, pp.81-2)

The question hinges upon the classical difference between a philosophical text and its preface, the preface usually being a recapitulation of the truth presented by the text. Since Derrida challenges the notion that a *text* can *present* a *truth*, his prefaces - in which this challenge is anticipated - must especially mark that which makes a text explode the classical ideas of truth and presence. And they must do so without letting the preface anticipate this 'conclusion' as a single, clear, luminous truth. Thus the *complication* of these prefaces. One way of complicating a preface is to leave as a knot that which will later become several strands.[4]

The preface should complicate rather than simplify. Not only must it not present the text as a single, clear, luminous truth, but it must not present the single, clear, luminous truth that it is *not* presenting the text as a single, clear, luminous truth. The preface must, of necessity, be duplicitous.

In this third preface the duplicity is taken literally; two interrelated, interleaved, entwined, cohabiting texts, neither of which can exist fully without the other, form a knot, a series of knots, of their several strands. You will see from the typeface in which they are written that I regard them both as con-text, as statements or theses in their own right, as attempts to refer to something in the world. I will leave you to decide the extent to which each is also a sub-text to the other; that is, to decide just who is scribbling in whose margin. I will also leave it to you to decide whether to read

'It is impossible to say which one quotes the other, and above all which one forms the border of the other. Each includes the other, comprehends the other, which is to say that neither comprehends the other. Each "narrative" *[récit]* (and each occurrence of the word "narrative", each "narrative" in the narrative) is part of the other, makes the other a part (of itself), each "narrative" is at once larger and smaller than itself, includes itself without including (or comprehending) itself, identifies itself with itself, even as it remains utterly different from its homonym.' (Derrida - Living on: border lines, pp.99-100)

the two columns together *à la* John Barth, or to read each as a separate text.

Notes

1 Derrida, J. (1979) Living on: border lines. In P. Kamuf (ed) *A Derrida Reader: Between the Blinds*, New York: Harvester Wheatsheaf, 1991, p.260
2 McLuhan, M. (1964) *Understanding Media*, London: Routledge, 2001, p.19
3 Ibid., p.21

4   Bass, A. Translator's introduction. In J. Derrida *Writing and Difference*, London: Routledge, 1978, pp.301-2

Losing the Plot	I Want to Write {Something} Different(ly)

And they all lived happily ever after. The End.

Narrative has a beginning, middle, and an end, but not necessarily in that order (Jean-Luc Godard 1971)

Where shall I start? The beginning, middle or end? It is usual when writing academic papers to begin with an abstract, that is to summarise the main points contained in the beginning, middle and end of the paper in a linear chronological framework. Interestingly, the abstract, which comes first, is usually written at the end of the paper, at which point the aim of the paper is deemed to have been achieved, but what if the purpose of the paper is the process?

Similarly, academic assignments usually require the student to say what they are going to say, to say it and then to say what they have said, thus revealing the plot a priori. This presupposes that a chronological framework exists in which this came after that which came after that and so on.

To audience: For the purpose

7 July
Dear Reader
I want to write something different. I would like us to have a discussion, a conversation. I would like us to talk about discourse. That is, I would like us to converse about:
(**dis**-korss) *n*. 1. A speech or lecture. 2. A written treatise on a subject.
(dis-**korss**) *v*. to utter or write a discourse[1]. So, I (almost) hear you saying, he wants to talk about talking, to write about writing, to dis-**korss** *v*. about **dis**-korss *n*. How very postmodern.

But no, that's not what I would like to do. In fact, my dictionary has no words, no definition, for the kind of discourse I want us to talk about, so instead, in this moment of crisis, I turn to a psychologist. He knows exactly what I want to discuss, he knows that I want us to explore 'a system of statements which construct an object'[2] (or, as Foucault[3] put it, 'a regulated practice that accounts for a number of statements').

A discourse is a discussion that a group of people, an academic community, a school, has with itself. This discourse, this discussion, this system of

of this paper I am not going to tell you what I am doing, to reveal the plot is to assume that there is one and that I know what it is. I don't know what it is (I don't think) ... exciting isn't it when you don't know where you are going to be taken ... or is it? But that is his story and another story altogether which I will tell you some other time...

When plotting the course of this paper I was wondering where to begin ... begin at the beginning but I am not sure where it is ... or even what it is ... perhaps it is in the middle ... so I'll start then with a procession:

'Ladies and Gentleman, perhaps you are going to listen ... you have, in any case, begun to hear. You are now hearing the first lines of a text ... the reading of the German translation of a text, written originally in French ...

Written then, not by me, the German announcer whose voice you hear...but by the French author, who speaks to you in my voice.

He has written this.

Or rather, if he were speaking himself, and, in reality, he is speaking to you himself, in my voice, he would say to you, he says to you: No I have not written this, I write, I am in the act of writing it, German listeners for you to hear.

I am in the act of writing

statements, engenders itself, creates an object out of itself that is its own discourse. Discourse is created through talk, and more importantly, through writing. A discourse is a way of talking and writing about the world (or part of it) that can only come about by talking or writing about the world (or part of it). A discourse is both a language and the objects of which that language speaks; both a practise and a practice. A discourse is (more or less) a language game, a game with its own rules and definitions; that is, 'a form of life'[4]. Most discourses are incompatible with most other discourses. Often they play very different language games. Often they fail to understand each other. Sometimes there is open hostility between them. Evidence-based practice is a discourse within most healthcare disciplines. So is reflective practice.

But perhaps I am starting at the wrong point. 'It is so difficult to find the beginning. Or better, it is difficult to begin at the beginning. And not try to go further back'[5]. So where to begin?

9 July

Dear Reader

I want to write differently. I am bored with writing academic papers, with always the same language game. I want to lose/loose/loosen this tired old plot. I want to translate my thoughts into a new language (game). I want to translate between discourses. Not to transliterate - that would be meaningless. No, I want to initiate 'an exercise in violent approximation'[6].

What is translation? On a platter
A poet's pale and glaring head,

these first lines. I am no more along in it than you. I am not more advanced than you. We are going to advance, are advancing already, together; you hearing, me speaking.

And yet, in fact, where am I? I am seated myself, at my table, in France, in my house. As for you, God knows where you are. You know well, yourself, where you are; you know it better than I. You know also if you are listening or only hearing, as you go about your business in your apartment and, perhaps even as you have some conversation, from here on I will pretend that you are listening to me....'[1].

This may come as a surprise but I didn't write this for this particular occasion, in fact I didn't write it at all, it was written by the French processual poet Francis Ponge. Ponge questions the notion of plot as we know it, as a poet he speaks of a new form of writing known as 'processual poetry'.

To Self: But will they get it, will they suss out the plot, that I am working reflexively or will I have to inadvertently reveal the plot and the meaning? I'll start like any good academic essay with the definitions.

Plot
    1.   A defined and usually
          small piece of ground

A parrot's screech, a monkey's chatter,
And profanation of the dead.
                          Vladimir Nabokov[7]

Nabokov wrote war poetry; the translator is a negotiator, a go-between in a continuous war between language (game)s. Jean-François Lyotard claimed that the job of the intellectual is to deny that this discourse war is taking place 'for the sake of political hegemony'[8]. An intellectual might be expected to say something like 'Describing the discussions and altercations of the past decade as a war paints the matter as more confrontational than necessary'[9]. It is therefore left to the philosopher to report on the war, to surface the disputes between different discourses and to 'find ... the (impossible) idiom for phrasing them'[10].

11 July
Dear Reader
I want to write {something} different(ly). I want to find the impossible idiom.

13 July
Dear Reader
I am writing this from a war zone; a war between discourses, a war over territory, a war between speakers of different languages, a war between creators of different realities, a war between different worlds.

A discipline is a world with limits, it is bounded by other disciplines. Sometimes a discipline is invaded by discourses from other disciplines, other worlds. Sometimes a discipline is at war with itself, a civil war between competing internal discourses.

A discipline is a world with limits, and

2. The interrelationship of the main events in a play, novel, film
3. A conspiracy or secret plan especially to achieve an unlawful end[2]

To self: I want a corner plot, Margaret and Colin, my neighbours, they live on a corner plot, they can see the view from all angles and importantly if anyone is plotting against them, they are in the neighbourhood watch scheme, scheme, that's another word for plot. Fran Biley has a plot of land, so did Arthur Fowler, he was in Eastenders, Guy Fawkes now that was a man with a plot. Films they have a plot, like that Sixth Sense, funny how we loved to be tricked, a twist in the tale reveals that Hermes is at play, we loved to be tricked in fiction but in real life control over the plot is important. Anything that wasn't part of the plan is seen as a nuisance. The Great Escape, a film that's always shown at Christmas, they thought they were to going to be free, but instead they were led to their death, films are not so good when you've seen them more than once, when you know the plot. So why is it that we watch the same films repeatedly even when we know the ending? Why was I asked here anyway?

territory is at a premium. Within a discipline:
1. Each discourse stakes its claim, claims its plot
2. Each discourse has a preferred way of relating its main events, of narrating its story; a more or less standard plot
3. Each discourse involves a secret plan, a conspiracy, a plot to protect its territory

15 July
Dear Jacques
Happy birthday (71 today)

17 July
Dear Reader
Every discourse has a narrative and a plot. The narrative is the story, the propaganda, that the discourse wishes to disseminate. The narrative is a story that is constructed in the telling. The writers are in the act of writing. They are no more along in it than you, the reader. They are not more advanced than you. They are going to advance, are advancing already, together; you reading, they writing.

Narrative has a beginning, middle, and an end, but not necessarily in that order. Some books, some films, begin by revealing the ending of the story, the ending of the plot. But that, after all, *is* the plot.

In others, the narrative steps outside of the plot (or does the plot step outside of the narrative?). Narrative is revealed as a plot, a trick, a conspiracy by the author, the director, to make us believe in a lie, the lie of the plot. *Blazing Saddles*, now there's a film with a plot. But all films have a plot, they plot to make you

To audience: Someone said my friend with Alzheimer's had lost the plot, I said what plot was that then…what does it mean when someone else has lost the plot…it means that the other person no longer behaves in a way which is congruent with the plot that I have written. Surely patients with Alzheimer's and Dementia have got another plot I said, one that we cannot access, they have only regressed if viewed within a linear timeframe, perhaps they have transgressed, transcended to a higher level of consciousness beyond our reach, where a different language is spoken, one that is pathologised, we try to cover the plot up rather than uncover it, cover it with normalizing routines and rituals, a plot that feels safe, one that we can follow, one that is socially constructed?

Whose plot is it that is lost, is there only one and if so who decides what it is?

Plot is surely socially constructed and can be deviated from, is plot the grand narrative that the individual deviates from in order to be individual? What is it to deviate from the plot?

'Alice is at an earlier stage of dementia than Fred. She is tubby but rather severe-looking with sunken eyes and sleeked back silvery hair. She can be

forget that you are watching a film, to make you believe that you are in a story, are part of the story (however far-fetched). You are so engaged in the narrative that you forget about the plot. The narrative is the juicy piece of meat carried by the burglar to distract the watchdog of the mind. You think that you are part of a cowboy story, until suddenly, without warning, you crash through the scenery and into a film lot. Or the *French Lieutenant's Woman*, where narrative and plot are completely entangled, and you don't know whether you are watching a Victorian love story, a film about a Victorian love story, or a film about making a film about a Victorian love story (or all three at once).

In attending to the narrative, we lose (forget) the plot. When we are made aware of the plot, the narrative begins to slip from our grasp.

Why am I writing this, anyway?

Is seeing the plot a form of transcendence? In losing the narrative, do we find the plot, the plot that the audience (being too preoccupied with the juicy piece of meat) rarely 'gets', rarely sees? It is said that in the kingdom of the blind, the one-eyed man is king. This is nonsense, of course. In the kingdom of the blind the one-eyed man is certified insane and locked up for speaking of a world (and often of a plot, of a conspiracy) that does not (empirically) exist for his fellows. You need only read Blake (and, by extension, Huxley and Laing) for confirmation:

How do you know but ev'ry Bird that cuts the airy way,
Is an immense world of delight, clos'd by your senses five?[11]

snappy and contentious. Sometimes she plods round singing 'her song' – "Hee-haw hee-haw…" with the volume turned up in a manner calculated to annoy. If you ask her why she does it she says, "I'm meaning mind your own business. But why don't you stop me doing it?"

Today she is in a pensive mood. "My memory has gone. And my hearing. I'll end up dotty. I'm afraid they'll break me up for firewood. I'm good for nothing else"[3] .

To self: But I diversify, the plot thickens … wonder if I can uncover it … now where shall I start.

A theoretical framework, that's what they want, a framework within which the plot can be lost, will that be a tragedy, comedy, satire, romance?

To audience: Narrative

To self: This is what they want

To audience: It is important to make a distinction between the notion of story, narrative and the concept of a plot.

Narrative is generating a great deal of interest in health related disciplines and appeals to the masses because it functions so readily as a focus for anti-positivist analyses of medical interventions. As such it is ripe for appropriation, research-

And later:

If the doors of perception were cleansed every thing would appear to man as it is, Infinite[12].

Or as R.D. Laing puts it in the opening gambit of his book *Knots*:

They are playing a game. They are playing at not playing a game. If I show them I see they are, I shall break the rules and they will punish me. I must play their game, of not seeing I see the game[13].

19 July
Dear Reader
My memory has gone. I can no longer follow the narrative. But I get the plot. I have smashed through the scenery. I can see the game.

23 July
Dear Reader
A theoretical framework; is that what you want? A template for constructing the plot. The golden rules for successful writing, the ten commandments that purify the discourse, written on tablets of stone:

Thou shalt base all thy practice on evidence;
Thou shalt not overgeneralise thy findings;
Thou shalt write clearly and concisely at all times;
and so on.

The plot: a plot to keep the discourse pure, so that 'madmen, charlatans, fakers, and sophists [especially sophists] are hopefully excluded from the ranks'[14];

ers and practitioners using the narrative approach need to ensure that if narrative and story are to become a 'genuine focus for nursing inquiry', then it is important that the meaning of these concepts is adequately defined and delimited[4]. Currently little, if any, distinction between the terms 'story' and 'narrative' in the context of healthcare, where it is used interchangeably.

According to Frank the difference between story and narrative is that story is a relational activity which takes place within a fluid social context and ethical matrix. Whereas narrative is more sophisticated and structured than a story, stories and tales are casual, informal and contingent. Narratives, he argues, are premeditated, organized and have a structure which is their own. The distinction then is that narratives contain a reflective or theoretical component involving meditation and contemplation. Frank offers a clear insight into the subtle differences between narrative and story in saying that 'The subtle semantics of narrative suggest a structure underpinning the story, and narrative analysis locates the structures that storytellers rely on but are not fully aware of'[5]. Wiltshire makes a clear distinction not only between story and narrative but also between these and the notions of expla-

a plot to keep the madmen out of our territory, off our plot; a simple narrative to distract us from the plot, to quieten the watchdog of the mind.

> Scientific education ... has the purpose of carrying out a rationalistic simplification of the process 'science' by simplifying its participants.... An essential part of that training is the inhibition of intuitions that might lead to a blurring of boundaries.... His imagination is restrained and even his language [game] will cease to be his own[15].

Or:

> Concern with method also stultifies the individual, dampens his strongest passions, and molds him to the requirements for membership in the scientific community. Most of all, however, correct method may block him from confronting experience and restricting his imagination. It limits possibility, it prevents him from realising what might have been....[16]

A plot to obscure the doors of perception, to prevent you from crashing through the scenery and out into the film lot, into the airy way.

24 July
Dear Reader
The narrative of positivism. Or should I say 'postpositivism'? But is a postpositivism even conceivable when 'The positive philosophy represents the true final state of human intelligence'[17]? But what, then, is this positivism, this positive philosophy? In what does it consist?

nation and account, the latter two being more closely aligned with power and authority. He discusses the concept of story and narrative and its relationship to other concepts such as explanation and account, arguing that story and narrative are different from account and explanation by the nature of the fact that they tend to imply a democracy of equals. Explanation, he argues, usually suggests that one person has more knowledge than the other.

The narrator, in contrast to the storyteller, selects and arranges material, participating by means of implicit reflection on the information and events being described. Narrative is thus: 'a reflective practice, whereas story is not. And because it is a reflective practice, narrative is connected, as story is not, with authority'[6]. This link with authority is significant given my earlier reference to power and autonomy, and has implications for who is writing/reading the narrative. Narration then is part of a reflective self-conscious and an interventionary process which requires abstract thought. It is integrational, requiring energy and intellectual and physical commitment.

The plot is the basic means by which specific events are brought into one meaningful whole[7]. That is to say that the

We have seen that the fundamental character of the positive philosophy is to consider all phenomena as subject to invariable natural laws. The exact discovery of these laws and their reduction to the least possible number constitute the goal of all our efforts; for we regard the search after what are called causes, whether first or final, as absolutely inaccessible and unmeaning[18].

To discover the 'invariable natural laws', but not to concern ourselves with their causes, which are 'absolutely inaccessible and unmeaning'. Positivism, then, is concerned only with the search for *evidence* of the operation of these laws in 'observed facts'.

Thus, to cite the best example, we say that the general phenomena of the universe are explained - as far as they can be - by the Newtonian law of gravitation. On the one hand, this admirable theory....[19]

Stop! Stop! Hasn't he read Einstein? Doesn't he know that 'The laws of the mechanics of Galilei-Newton can be regarded as valid only for a Galileian system of co-ordinates'[20]? But how could he, since he was writing fifty years before Einstein was born. I repeat, dear Reader: *How could Comte have known about Einstein's partial refutation of Newton's 'admirable theory' when he died fifty years before it was published?* But that, of course, is the whole point. Comte's 'positive philosophy' was based on 'the precepts of Bacon, the conceptions of Descartes, and the discoveries of Galileo'[21]. It was, in a nutshell, an induc-

plot is the structure underpinning the story, which as Frank suggests may or may not be conscious. Enplotment is the central process in narrative providing order and meaning to the previous chaotic flow of events, from this a configuration of succession procession is derived[8]. Enplotment is not a finished event but an ongoing process, as new information arises the plot is accordingly adjusted, thus it is a dynamic process which is always in the process of becoming[9]. The basic modernist narrative has a beginning, middle and end. The beginning introduces the participants, the middle describes the main action sequences and the end describes the consequences[10]. Northrop Frye[11], who actually coined the term enplotment, identified four archetypal plot structures: comedy, romance, tragedy, and satire. These plots have been discussed in the context of wider life.

Brooks[12] suggests we both create narratives and are created by them; they are part of our very being. They bring order to disorder, but I would argue that disorder itself is a narrative with its own plot, which in turn gives order to disorder. The reflective practitioner, like the researcher, in their desire to avoid too much uncertainty can move too quickly to order and premature closure or end-

tive philosophy, a systematic collection and categorisation of evidence, part of a continuing narrative story that began in the sixteenth century and whose ending no one could anticipate. No matter how admirable the theory, there is always the possibility of some Einstein coming along tomorrow, next week, or in fifty years, and rewriting the ending. And ultimately, of course, the same fate befell Comte's own 'great fundamental law'[22] that positivism is the 'true final state of human intelligence'.

Being itself based on induction, then, the law of the true final state of human intelligence proved not to be, and 'the naive positivist position of the sixteenth through the nineteenth centuries is no longer held by anyone even casually acquainted with these problems'[23]. Thus, 'the postpositivist position represents an attempt to transform positivism in ways that take account of these same objections'[24]. Recognising that the inductive search for positive evidence can never prove a theory, the postpositivists turned instead to Popper's falsificationism which recognised that, although we can never *prove* a theory it is nevertheless a simple matter to *disprove* it. So, if we reject the search for first causes and collect only evidence of the *effects* of first causes, we can never prove Newton's law of gravity (what goes up must come down), since we can never be certain that, tomorrow, a particular apple might just keep going up. But, of course, if that apple *does* just go up, then we have, at a stroke, refuted the theory.

25 July
Dear Reader
I seem to have lost my place. Where

ing. Through the telling of stories we intensify and clarify the plot structure of events as lived, eliminating events that in retrospect are not important to the development of that plot, which do not as we say contribute to the ending. But as Murray has already pointed out the notion of an ending is in itself a narrative by which to order our experience. Reflective narratives may be full of purpose without knowing what it is that they, the reflective practitioner, are tending towards; their purpose is not manifest as a clearly framed goal, more likely a troubling, as in the discomfort that spurs the practitioner into a reflective process. The fate of the narrative though is not sealed (from the past) but signified in the emerging plot. A narrative then is created through a person's narration, as is the narrator.

In telling their stories, the narrators shape their narratives to the audience. Storytellers always require a cast of listeners, for the client it is the nurses, for the practitioner it is the client and others, for me it is you. Narrators can exaggerate certain elements of the story or downplay other aspects. The character of the relationship between the two partners in guided reflection is of vital importance in this interplay of connecting conversations. Importantly then storytelling is

was I? Oh yes, the narrative of postpositivism. Postpositivist science recognises its own impotence, accepts that nothing can be proven. It is therefore impelled to reveal the *dénouement* of its narrative in the very first line; the hypothesis; 'a fictive beginning, a false exit'[25]; a happy ending that can never be. Like a film plot revealed in a series of flashbacks, the narrative of postpositivist scientific research begins at the end before meticulously working its way back to that predetermined conclusion.

In order to make generalisations, to tell the story of everyone, the narrative of scientific research is decontextualised, devoid of specific characters in specific settings. The narrative of scientific research is thus a story told by nobody about no one, who lives nowhere. The story is not set anywhere in the world, but it refers to everywhere in the world. The story is not about anyone, but it refers to everyone. The story has no narrator but (usually) several authors who pretend that they had no influence over the unfolding drama, who pretend that they were not present as the drama was enacted.

> Because it begins by repeating itself, such an event at first takes the form of a story. Its first time takes place several times. Of which, one, among others, is the last. Numerous and plural in every strand of its (k)nots (that is, (k)not any subject, (k)not any object, (k)not any thing), this first time already is not from around here, no longer has a here and now; it breaks up the complicity of belonging that ties us to our habitats, our culture, our simple roots[26].

for another just as much as it is for oneself. Here one could easily substitute nursing for guided reflection. For narrative practitioners do not regard conversations as expressions of meaning, but rather as the sites where meaning is created in people's lives. Conversations do not only describe experience; they generate experience and are both unique in the moment and limited by the cultural assumptions and possibilities of their contexts. Narratives then as acts of telling 'are relationships'[13]. The risk of reducing the story to a narrative is that of 'losing the purpose for which people engage in storytelling' which Frank argues is relationship building. This perhaps fits with Ricoeur's sense of narrative and its relationship to life. Life he says can be seen as 'an activity and a passion in search of a narrative'[14]. This begs some interesting questions regarding the notion of research ethics in narrative inquiry, which are relational and relationship and come before method; one cannot ever analyse a relationship without entering into it, more knowledge may be less important than a sense of clearer value and authentic truth. What is the relationship between narrative inquiry (and guided reflection) and authentic truth and value?

Why all this talk of (k)nots, of 'tangles, fankles, *impasses*, disjunctions, whirligogs, binds'[27]?

27 July
Dear Reader
Popper (perhaps naively) believed that he had solved the problem of induction: rather than collect positive evidence to *prove* theories, science should be concerned with setting up hypotheses which we then attempt to *disprove*[28]. Thus:

Hypothesis H_1:
What goes up must come down
Null hypothesis H_0:
What goes up does not come down

Since it is impossible to prove H_1, we should concern ourselves rather with disproving H_0, that is, by designing experiments that deliberately set out to find a situation in which an apple will *not* come down. The more rigorous our tests, the stronger will be the theory that survives them.

Postpositivist scientific evidence, then, is purely negative; it consists in demonstrating what is *not* the case, or rather, in showing that there is no evidence to support the null hypothesis. Strictly speaking, then (and we must, of course, speak strictly), the evidence *for* a particular practice is actually a *lack* of evidence *against* it. When the postpositivists claim to have proved that a particular practice is effective, they have, in truth, merely failed to prove that it is ineffective. Let's take another example. It is impossible to collect enough evidence to prove that a certain drug is safe. First, however many rats, dogs, people it is tested on, there is always the possibility of an adverse reac-

To self: Now I'm really cooking, this will keep them happy.

Narrative Inquiry

To audience: According to Josselson and Lieblich narrative research is 'a process of inquiry that embraces paradox and cannot therefore be defined in linear terms'[15]. It is cyclical and always in the process of becoming. Narrative analysis is not designed to make a new plot or new meaning, although this will inevitably occur should the research be reflexive, but to expose the limitations and constraints of old meanings and old plots. Many writers who emphasize the modality of narrative argue that all truth is 'constructed' and therefore local and contingent. There is not one knowledge or truth, but a variety of competing 'knowledges' each of which is developed within a specific cultural, professional or institutional framework. Emphasising the 'fictive' provisional and discursive aspects of all 'knowledge production', they draw on such sources as Kuhn's work on scientific paradigms and Foucault to dispute the outright truth claims of science. Postmodern theorists argue that narrative is already woven into the fabric of science; for example science itself is a story[16]. The notion of truth therefore that goes along with narrative (and guided reflection) is that of it

tion on someone (anyone) who was not part of the trial. Second, however long the trial lasted, there is always the possibility of delayed side-effects becoming apparent tomorrow, next week, in fifty years. The best that science can do is to fail to prove that the drug is harmful. The failure to confirm a null hypothesis (this drug has harmful side-effects) is the best that science can offer us. Postpositivism is more correctly negativism, and evidence-based practice depends entirely on an absence of evidence.

30 July
Dear Reader

I am beginning to realise why the post-positivists are so aggressive in their promotion of evidence-based practice. What would Freud have said? Overcompensation? Reaction formation? Or perhaps penis envy? When they shout loudly for more evidence it is because they know that evidence-based practice depends, precisely, on a lack. When they condemn practice based on other criteria it is because they know, at heart, that they have no evidence to prove their own practice.

You think I am overstating the case, I can tell. Well, then, let's look at a case to see whether it is overstated; let's look at the case of Raymond Tallis and his paper 'Evidence-based and evidence-free generalisations: a tale of two cultures'[29].

1 August
Dear Reader

Where to start? I suppose at the beginning, with the title. *A tale of two cultures*, a reference to C.P. Snow I imagine: culture wars; art *versus* science. For Tallis:

being local and contingent and constructed in relation[17]. This notion of relational truth is linked to the practice of co-operative inquiry and has implications for the understanding and experiencing of power and authority.

Co-operative inquiry is a systematic approach to developing understanding and action, and involves what Reason and Heron call an 'extended epistemology'[18], that is it extends beyond the primarily theoretical knowledge of academia to include many different ways of knowing. The researcher claims, inevitably and often effectively, to be the master of the code that makes some underlying phenomenon intelligible. That code may be termed any number of things, but analysts who identify the code underlying some social order unavoidably present themselves as the masters of that order. The auspices of this knowing as mastery is often called a methodology[19]. These methodological codes describe some aspects of social life and are useful in their own way, indeed I have used and continue to use them myself. Nevertheless, one needs to view this whole issue of methodology and mastery of the data with suspicion when referring to the concept of co-operative inquiry and in the development of narrative

a   the purpose of academic study, of scholarship, is to express truths about the world in general;
b   all expressions of truth must be supported by evidence;
c   evidence must be collected rigorously and 'scientifically', preferably using the method of the randomised controlled trial.

Now, when Tallis is discussing medicine, this is a reasonable set of assumptions, although his assertion that 'The only truly robust method for obtaining good evidence is the double-blind randomised controlled trial' is perhaps already beginning to sound dated, and even extreme. Nevertheless, as I said, it is a reasonable set of assumptions.

The problem, however, is that Tallis does not wish to restrict his criteria for good scholarship simply to medicine, nor indeed simply to science. Literary theory, he claims, has run into problems because of 'the lack of *appropriate quantitative methods* to acquire the data necessary to underpin descriptive general statements and to ensure the validity of causal explanations' (my italics). Tallis is happy enough for individual scholars to beaver away with 'close readings' of individual texts, so long as they don't have the temerity to make pronouncements about the wider world. They can, if they wish, 'argue forcefully over the interpretation of a particular word in *Hamlet*', but are not entitled to widen their scope to discussions 'about the nature of society, the relationship between language and the world, the origin of the self, the interaction between knowledge and power, and so forth', due to 'the minute size of the database upon which such statements are

approaches. There are of course a number of issues regarding the rigour of such reflexive approaches, these will not be elaborated upon here, suffice it to say that I agree with other authors and researchers who argue a position on goodness that holds that the product of inquiry should serve the community studied, rather than one's discipline.

Recently narrative is generating so much interest in health related disciplines and appeals to the masses because it functions so readily as a focus for anti-positivist analyses of medical interventions, it is ripe for appropriation, need to ensure that if narrative and story are to become a 'genuine focus for nursing inquiry', then it is important that the meaning of these concepts is adequately defined and delimited. Currently little, if any, distinction between the term story and narrative in the context of healthcare, used interchangeably.

To self: Wonder if they will notice that I am repeating myself, will they get it? Perhaps they will be thinking I have heard this somewhere before, where was it? More likely they will think I have made a mistake and will be too polite to say so. Maybe they will think I am demented.

founded' (what was I saying earlier about penis envy?). But this 'evidence-free' or (at best) 'evidence poor' practice is not restricted to literary studies. No, 'the lack of appropriate quantitative methods... lies at the heart of the present crisis in *the humanities*' (my italics). Tallis continues: 'In an age in which it is increasingly expected that general statements should be supported by robust evidence if they are to command credence, the humanities are in danger of being simply anachronistic, *acceptable only to arts graduates who have known no better* and are unacquainted with adequate methodological discipline' (my italics). So there we have it. The arts, the humanities, even philosophy, wiped out with a single stroke of the pen. The final decisive battle in the culture wars.

But wait; Tallis throws a lifeline, there is still hope. 'What new approach will protect the humanities from the kind of charlatanry that, much to the disgust of many honest scholars, threatens to overwhelm it?'. He continues: 'Huge collaborative effort would be necessary to acquire data adequate to support the kinds of claims that are routinely made in cultural history and criticism'. Let's not get too excited, though, since 'While this effort is unquestionably worthwhile when one is evaluating a new treatment for a serious condition such as stroke, it may not be thought to be justified merely in order to establish some general truths of cultural history'. Ah yes, he anticipates, but 'Humanist academics often defend their data-poor assertions by suggesting that this would not only be difficult; it would also be inappropriate'. But then, what do they know, being only 'humanist academics' and specialists in their field.

To audience: 'The senior sister tells me some stories about Alice. The unit offers a secure and caring environment and certain necessary precautions are taken to prevent those who are confused from getting lost or endangering themselves. One day Alice comes up to her and poses the question "Tell me, is love the key?" to which the affirmative answer is given. Then comes the follow up "And do you love me?" Again an affirmative answer. Then the sharp retort "Well if love is the key, and you love me – why don't you open the bloody door?"'[20].

Wiltshire discusses the concept of story and narrative and its relationship to other concepts such as explanation and account, arguing that story and narrative are different from account and explanation by the nature of the fact that they tend to imply a democracy of equals. Explanation, he tells us, usually suggests that one person has more knowledge than the other.

The basic modernist narrative has a beginning, middle and end. The beginning introduces the participants: Did I say I am Dr Dawn Freshwater, what I'd like to talk about today is linked to the notion of a plot … and narrative … the middle describes the main action sequences and the end describes the consequences[21].

No, Tallis, the medical doctor (albeit with an honorary degree of Doctor of Letters), has the last word: 'I would argue that large-scale empirical statements - such as are made by many cultural theorists and historians - have to be underpinned by properly designed large-scale empirical enquiries'. Furthermore, 'If one does not have the means to acquire the data to support higher-level generalisations, one should avoid them. In short, if you can't substantiate statements, don't make them'.

So, in a nutshell:

a   the humanities will only gain academic credibility by generating rigorous, large scale, empirical evidence from quantitative studies;

b   such an endeavour would require enormous and probably unobtainable resources;

c   in any case, the end result would not be worth the effort;

d   the humanities are thus condemned to remain unsubstantiated and therefore inconsequential, suitable only for the interpretation of a particular word in *Hamlet*.

3 August
Dear Reader

Do you still think I am overstating my case; that there isn't at least a little overcompensation at work? Or perhaps you are thinking that maybe Tallis has a point. Let me tell you why I think not; evidence, if you like, although not the kind of evidence to which Tallis would give credence.

Evidence; or lack of evidence. Consider: if Tallis is right in his claim that we may not make general claims about the world without adequate quantitative

To self: Is this reflexive satire?

To audience: Narrative analysis is not designed to make a new plot or new meaning (although this will inevitably occur should the research be reflexive) but expose the limitations and constraints of old meanings and old plots.

Whatever your definition of reflexivity, one cannot avoid the fact that it essentially involves the subjective self, and the ability of the self to turn back on itself. This is important in the context of both reflective inquiry and reflexive research, that is the uncovering of the plot, for as Bentz and Shapiro comment 'Research is always carried out by an individual with a life and a *lifeworld,* a personality, a social context, and various personal and practical challenges and conflicts, all of which affect the research, from the choice of a research question or topic, through the method used, to the reporting of the project's outcome'. They go on to say that 'the very act of posing a research question will shape and influence the answer'[22]. Or as Paris prefers 'Wherever there is a Narrator (and how could there not be?), there is no objective biography, no more than objective history …'[23]. The narrator (researcher/guide) is part of the process of transforming practice and is in the same instance transform-

evidence, then he is also wrong in his claim, which is, of course, made without adequate quantitative evidence; indeed, without any evidence whatsoever. Or as Laing would say:

JILL   You put me in the wrong
JACK I am not putting you in the wrong
JILL   You put me in the wrong for
        thinking you put me in the wrong[30]

When Tallis accuses his opponents of not producing evidence for their assertions, he means hard, quantitative empirical evidence derived from 'properly designed large-scale empirical enquiries'. So, Derrida cannot be trusted since 'much of what he says is unsupported by evidence'. Worse still, Derrida sometimes distorts what little evidence he has. How do we know this? Well, says Tallis, 'There is prima facie evidence' that it is so. Furthermore, 'There is evidence that these errors are systematic'. Given Tallis's earlier pronouncements on evidence, we might expect that this 'evidence' is derived from 'properly designed large-scale empirical enquiries'. But no, 'it is interesting to note that this distortion had to be pointed out by a non-academic and was published, not in a scholarly journal but in a literary weekly - *The Times Literary Supplement*. Not only was the 'evidence' not empirically based, it was not produced by an academic and not published in a scholarly journal. It is, perhaps, pushing at the limits of credibility to see how, by Tallis's reckoning, it is evidence at all.

But Tallis is not so blind that he cannot see this objection himself: 'I am uncomfortably aware that I am not above this process as I write the present chapter....

ed, it is therefore not possible for them to be available in a therapeutic manner whilst being concerned with the process of phenomenological 'bracketing'.

When we tell stories we intensify and clarify the plot structure of events as lived, eliminating events that in retrospect are not important to the development of that plot, which do not as we say contribute to the ending, but the notion of an ending is in itself a narrative by which to order our experience, perhaps the ending is already written and we live our lives accordingly, illness narratives, genetic/hereditary illness, how does this link to health promotion and the concept of prevention, prevention of what ... a plot that is already written or a plot that will write us ... if we are not careful.

To self: Is this what we mean when we say take care? The plot will get you; the plot is out there!

To audience: But, *my English teacher always taught me to say however as I am more likely to get the person I am speaking to on my side.* Narrative practitioners do not regard conversations as expressions of meaning, but rather as the sites where meaning is created in people's lives, conversations do not only describe experience;

which has been anecdote-driven and dependent upon a selection of quotations from primary and secondary sources. However, *so long as my comments are understood as the first word and not the last, this may be acceptable'* (my italics).

So that's OK then. Barthes, Lacan, Derrida and all the other writers that Tallis takes to task as being 'evidence-free' were attempting to have the final word on the matter, whereas Tallis was having the first word, was initiating an open-ended discussion. 'In short, if you can't substantiate statements, don't make them', says Tallis. A first word? If so, then what is the reply, and how is such a reply to be substantiated? I can think of few words more final, especially since Tallis also pointed out that 'properly' substantiated replies (that is, evidence-based replies) are almost impossible to make in the arts and humanities.

So what of Derrida *et al*, the writers accused by Tallis of having the final word? If you have read this far, dear Reader, you will perhaps know better, you will perhaps know that Derrida's project is not to shut down dialogue but to open it up: 'For there *must* not be a last word - that's what I'd like to say finally; the *afterword* is not, that means *ought* not, ought never to be a last word'[31]. The whole, entire, complete project of deconstruction is to open up the text to multiple readings, whereas the project of evidence-based practice is, on the whole, to arrive at a single 'correct' prescription for each and every problem. But perhaps I am in danger of overstating my own case. Let us just say, then, that it is by no means clear that Tallis means simply to have the first word

they generate experience and are both unique in the moment and limited by the cultural assumptions and possibilities of their contexts. Reading of writing is also a two-way process.

Storytelling is for another just as much as it is for oneself, reciprocity of the story, the moral genius of storytelling is that each, teller and listener, enters the space of the story for the other. One example of this is biography, did you know Winnicott's, (the British psychoanalyst), biography begins with the words 'I died' and is shortly followed with ... 'let me see what was happening when I died' ... he goes on to confirm that he was alive when he died.

To self: Life...death, what do they mean? How do I put together into a coherent image the pieces of my life? Even the notion of coherence presupposes a plot.

To audience: Life already has a plot, we trim a life to fit the frame, like a CV, an itinerary which tells you where you have been before you get there. The course of your life has been described in the future perfect tense. What is a CV if not a plot, a biographical one, but itemizing events for a resumé organized only by chronology (this came after that) - such a life is a narrative without a plot, its

in an ongoing debate, nor that Derrida *et al* intend to have the last word. But more importantly, being 'understood as the first word' is hardly sufficient justification for us to excuse Tallis from his own critique.

It is all too easy to play Tallis at his own (language) game, and his paper is perhaps an unwitting demonstration (proof, if you like) of Derrida's assertion that texts deconstruct themselves (some, albeit, more readily than others). But despite the simplicity with which Tallis's paper simply falls apart at the slightest tug of a loose thread, a stronger objection is surely that he has simply missed the point. The reason that the culture war is intractable is that (for the reasons I have just demonstrated) it cannot be fairly fought on the territory of either party. We have just seen what happens when the scientists are playing at home, and something equally horrible occurs when the artists are waging war on *their* own ground (you need look no further than Socal and Bricmont's book *Intellectual Impostures*[32] for some excellent and at times hilarious examples of social theorists attempting to write science).

4 August
Dear Reader
Am I losing the plot? Oh, yes, we were talking about missing the point. Tallis has, I would argue, simply missed the point, lost the plot. Art, science and philosophy are simply telling different stories using different language games. It is sometimes difficult even to communicate *within* these broad disciplines (witness the disputes between quantitative and qualitative scientists, between figurative and expressionist painters and between

focus on a more and more boring central figure that is 'me' wandering in the desert of dried out 'experiences'. What is the end purpose of this life? To what intended ends do we live? Is the plot the means to the end?

Narrative practitioners need to distinguish between Telos and teleology. Teleology indicates events are pulled by a purpose to a definite end, Telos, meaning end or fulfilment, which is not the same as causality which asks who started it, asking what initiated a motion, imagining events pushed from behind by the past. Teleology asks what's the purpose, conceiving events aimed towards a plot whose purpose is not always clear. The pull of purpose comes with force, Telos is full of purpose without knowing what it is and how to get there, not relying on a clearly framed goal, more likely a troubling, unclear urge coupled with a sense of indubitable importance.

'On another occasion Alice, who is a staunch Methodist, says "I have been thinking. I feel that after meals everyone should be upstanding for the Lord to thank him for all his loving kindnesses and for the lovely meal we have consumed."

"Well then" says the Sister, "Why don't you get up after the

analytic and postmodern philosophers) and communication across them is guaranteed to tie everyone involved in (k)nots.

For example, Richard Rorty distinguished between two philosophies:

> The first tradition takes scientific truth as the center of philosophical concern (and scorns the notion of incommensurable scientific world pictures). It asks how well other fields of inquiry conform to the model of science. The second tradition takes science as one (not especially privileged nor interesting) sector of culture, a sector which, like all other sectors, only makes sense when viewed historically. The first likes to present itself as a straightforward, down-to-earth, scientific attempt to get things right. The second needs to present itself obliquely, with the help of as many foreign words and as much allusiveness and name dropping as possible[33].

On this reading, Tallis and Derrida are representatives of the two philosophies, engaged in different projects with different aims, and using different languages with no chance of finding any common ground. As Derrida observed at the end of an exchange with another writer from the 'first philosophy':

> I ask myself if we will ever be quits with this confrontation.
> Will it have taken place, this time? Quite?[34]

So, I (almost) hear you say, what then is the point of this book? Aren't you simply

next meal and lead us all in a little prayer?"

And so after supper, Alice takes the lead "Everybody stand ..." and the prayer is a lovely one. The only problem is that al ten minute intervals throughout the following three hours the voice comes "Everybody stand ..." and the whole ritual is repeated ad infinitum. Alice is predictable only in her unpredictability'[24].

A narrative Is created through a person's narration. According to Ricoeur, narration means an activity where the interesting aspect is 'the activity that produces plots', rather than the plot itself[25].

The narrative contains a direction (directedness) that makes its wholeness into something greater than its parts[26]. This direction depends on the narrator's narrative skill[27]. Ricoeur[28] describes this as an ability to formulate narrative sentences and join them into a coherent narrative, where the parts are related to each other, contributing towards an explanation with the help of a plot.

I'd like to start my paper by processing through the text and reading a poem:

It's so foolish getting in a knot,
or grieving about getting in a knot.
I want to get to the point

another Tallis, a Tallis in reverse, a Sillat, applying the philosophical narrative of deconstruction to the scientific narrative of evidence-based practice?

Well, yes, but my (paradoxical) intention is to cross the boundaries between discourses, between disciplines, in order to show how it is often *impossible* to do so, to show how evidence-based practice simply deconstructs itself as soon as it leaves its natural home of testing medications. I am attempting to write as a philosopher (as Lyotard put it) rather than as an intellectual, and after all, the job of philosophy is to expose the schisms, the fractures, the *aporia* that become immediately apparent when a language game from one narrative is imposed on an incompatible one. If not finding the impossible idiom, than at least pointing out that, perhaps, there is no *possible* idiom, no true and accurate translation. As Hélèn Cixous observed: 'I have thought certain mysteries In the French language that I cannot think in English. This loss and this gain are in writing too'[35].

6 August
Dear Reader
Why all this talk of (k)nots? Perhaps I should leave the last word to Laing[36]:

the proposition
    'All forms point to the formless'
is itself a formal proposition
Not,
    as finger to moon
    so form to formless
but,
    as finger to moon
    so

Where it's a case of a matter of
course.
After all, what is this lump
Of matter if you can't make
sense of it.

All possible expressions, forms,
propositions, including this one,
made or yet to be made,
together with the brackets

are to

7 August
Dear Reader
I seem to have lost my pen...

I seem to have lost my place
... ahhh here it is

Notes

1   Ponge, F. *Soap*. California:
    Stanford University Press,
    1969 p.7
2   *Oxford English Dictionary*.
    Oxford: OUP,1996
3   Killick, J. *Please give me
    back my personality*.
    University of Stirling:
    Scotland, 1994, p.2
4   Wiltshire, J. Telling a story,
    writing a narrative:
    terminology in healthcare.
    Nursing Inquiry 1995, 2, 75-
    82
5   Frank, A.W. The Standpoint
    of Storyteller. *Qualitative
    Health Research*, 2000,
    May, p.354-365
6   Wiltshire, op. cit.
7   Abma, T.A. Powerful Stories:
    The role of stories in
    sustaining and transforming
    professional practice within
    a mental health hospital. In
    Josselson, R. and Lieblich, A.
    (Eds) *Making Meaning of
    Narratives*. California: Sage,
    1999, ch7
8   Ricoeur, P. *Hermeneutics
    and the human sciences*

Notes

1   *Oxford Paperback Dictionary*, Oxford:
    OUP, 1988
2   Parker, I. *Discourse Dynamics: Critical
    Analysis for Social and Individual
    Psychology*, London: Routledge,
    1992, p.5
3   Foucault, M. (1969) *The Archaeology
    of Knowledge*, London: Tavistock,
    1972, p.80
4   Wittgenstein, L. (1953) *Philosophical
    Investigations*, Oxford: Basil Blackwell,
    1972, para 19
5   Wittgenstein, L. *On Certainty*, Oxford:
    Blackwell, 1974, para. 471
6   Johnson, B. Translator's introduction. In
    J. Derrida (1972) *Dissemination*,
    London: Athlone, 1981, p.xviii
7   Nabokov, V. On translating "Eugene
    Onegin", cited in Derrida, ibid., p.vii
8   Lyotard, J.-F. (1983) *The Differend:
    Phrases in Dispute*, Minneapolis:
    University of Minnesota Press, 1988,
    p.142
9   Guba, E.G. & Lincoln, Y.S. Competing
    paradigms in qualitative research. In
    N.K. Denzin & Y.S. Lincoln (eds) *The
    Landscape of Qualitative Research*,
    Thousand Oaks: Sage, 1998, p.218
10 Lyotard, op. cit., p.142
11 Blake, W. (1790) *The Marriage of*

(Thompson, J.B. ed/trans),
Cambridge University Press:
Cambridge, 1981

9   Parse, R.R. *Nursing Science:
    major paradigms, theories
    and critiques.* Philadelphia:
    Saunders, 1987

10 Murray, M. The storied
    nature of health and illness.
    In Murray, M. and
    Chamberlain, K. (Eds.)
    *Qualitative Health
    Psychology.* London: Sage,
    1999

11 Frye, N. *Anatomy of
    Criticism.* Princeton:
    Princeton University Press,
    1957

12 Brooks, P. *Reading for the
    plot, design and intention in
    narrative.* Harvard: Harvard
    University Press, 1984

13 Frank op. clt.p.354

14 Ricoeur, P. *From Text to
    Action. Essays in
    Hermeneutics, II.*
    Northwestern University Press:
    Evanston, 1991, p.29

15 Josselson, R. and Lieblich, A.
    (Eds) *Making Meaning of
    Narratives.* California: Sage,
    1999

16 Lyotard, J-P. *The
    Postmodern condition: A
    report on knowledge.*
    Manchester University Press:
    Manchester, 1984

17 Wiltshire, op. cit.

18 Reason, P. and Heron, J. *A
    laypersons guide to co-
    operative inquiry.*
    http://www.bath.ac.uk/carp
    p/layguide/htm 1989, p3

Heaven and Hell, Oxford: OUP, 1975,
p.xvii

12 Ibid., p.xxii

13 Laing, R.D. (1970) *Knots*,
    Harmondsworth: Penguin, 1972, p.1

14 Phillips, D.L. *Abandoning Method*, San
    Francisco: Jossey Bass, 1973, p.154

15 Feyerabend, P.K. Against method:
    outline of an anarchistic theory of
    knowledge, *Minnesota Studies in the
    Philosophy of Science*, 1970, 4, 17-
    130, p.20

16 Phillips, op. cit., pp. 156-7

17 Comte, A. (1830) *Introduction to
    Positive Philosophy*, Indianapolis:
    Hackett, 1988, p.7

18 Ibid., p.8

19 Ibid., p.8

20 Einstein, A. (1916) *Relativity*, London:
    Routledge, 2001, p.13

21 Comte, op. cit., p.11

22 Ibid., p.1

23 Guba & Lincoln, op. cit., p.218

24 Ibid., p.218

25 Derrida, J. (1972) *Dissemination*,
    London: Athlone, 1981, p.305

26 Ibid., p.292

27 Laing, op. cit.

28 Popper, K.R. (1971) Conjectural
    knowledge: my solution to the
    problem of induction. In K.R. Popper,
    Objective Knowledge, Oxford:
    Clarendon Press, 1979

29 Tallis, R. Evidence-based and
    evidence-free generalisations: a tale
    of two cultures. In M. Grant (ed) *The
    Raymond Tallis Reader*, Basingstoke:
    Palgrave, 2000. All the following
    unreferenced citations are from this
    essay

30 Laing, op. cit., p.21

31 Derrida, J. Afterw.rds or, at least, less
    than a letter about a letter less. In N.

19 Frank, op. cit.
20 Killick, op. cit., p.4
21 Murray, op. cit.
22 Bentz, V.M. and Shapiro, J. *Mindful Inquiry in Social Research,* California: Sage, 1995, p.1
23 Paris, G. Pagan Grace. *Woodstock:* Spring 1995
24 Killick, op. cit., p2
25 Ricoeur, P. *Time and Narrative, 1.* The University of Chicago Press: Chicago, 1984, p. 33
26 Riceour 1991, op. cit.
27 Frid, I., Ohlen, J. & Bergbom, I. On the use of narratives in nursing education. *Journal of Advanced Nursing* 2000, 32 (3), 695-703
28 Riceour 1991, op. cit.

Royle (ed) *Afterwords*, Tampere: Outside Books, 1992, p.197
32 Socal, A. & Bricmont, J. *Intellectual Impostures*, London: Profile Books, 1998
33 Rorty, R. Philosophy as a kind of writing, *New Literary History*, 1978, X, 141-5, p.143
34 Derrida, J. Limited Inc. abc, *Glyph*, 1977, II, 162-254, p.251
35 Cixous, H. *Three Steps on the Ladder of Writing*, New York: Columbia University Press, 1993
36 Laing, op. cit., pp.87-8

Deconstruction

'Perhaps deconstruction has never done anything but ... interpret interpretation'
(Jacques Derrida - The Time is Out of Joint)

Deconstruction 1

Listen/read/write:
an exercise in deconstruction

... we must remain faithful, even if it implies a certain violence, to the injunctions of the text. These injunctions will differ from one text to the next so that one cannot prescribe one general method of reading. In this sense deconstruction is not a method.[1]

If deconstruction is not a method; if, as McQuillan suggests, 'there is no set of rules, no criteria, no procedure, no programme, no sequence of steps, no *theory* to be followed in deconstruction'[2], then how is it to be achieved? But if we accept McQuillan's description of deconstruction as 'an act of reading which allows the other to speak'[3], then it is 'a reading which is sensitive to what is irreducible in every text, allowing the text to speak before the reader, and listening to what the text imposes on the reader'[4]. Deconstruction, then, is more than an act of reading; it is an act of listening, of listening to the murmurings of the text, of listening to the hesitant stuttering whispers that can just be made out (if we listen attentively) below the confidently raised voice of the 'message' that the author wishes to convey.

McQuillan identifies two consequences of this view of deconstruction. First, 'deconstruction only *ever* happens once'[5]. It is a singular act, a one-off, it 'is not a thing [method] in this sense: it is a situation or an event of reading. Deconstruction is what happens'[6]. And what happens only *ever* happens once. Hence, each deconstructive reading is different, singular, unique, unreproducible.

Second, deconstruction (as we saw earlier) is impossible, since 'whenever we think we are hearing the other speak we are always reducing its otherness to the self-same'[7]. My deconstruction of a text is, in part, a deconstruction of myself, since the text speaks differently to me each time I read it.

It is therefore futile to attempt to offer a set of guidelines, or even a general strategy for deconstruction[8] other than to say: listen, and in particular, listen to what Roland Barthes calls the 'rustle of language', the 'grain' of the writing[9], the murmurings that occur in the margins, in the footnotes, in the jokey asides; listen carefully while the less discriminating reader is waiting impatiently for the 'message' to resume. And write; for if nothing else, 'deconstruction is not what you think'[10]; it is what you write.

What follows is a deconstruction, *my* deconstruction, of one of the seminal works of evidence-based medicine, indeed, of *the* seminal work (in the literal sense that it sowed the seeds for the entire movement). I had two reasons for choosing this paper: first, as the original statement of evidence-based medicine, it has a certain importance to the movement; and second, it is not necessary to listen particularly attentively in order to hear the contradictions, the *aporias* in the message, since they speak almost as loudly as the message itself. You might object, then, that I have taken unfair advantage of the text, that it is an infant (literally, as one of Derrida's translators pointed out, without voice[11]) whose babblings would be refined as it grew and discovered more about itself. Perhaps, but you will see from the wider deconstruction of evidence-based practice in *Deconstruction 2* that this is not the case, that evidence-based practice has grown from a confused and uncertain baby into a confused and uncertain young man (for it is surely not a woman).

You will find the original paper (con-text) reproduced in the left hand column and a deconstruction (sub-text) entitled *The Annunciation* in the right hand column. You will also find that my deconstructive sub-text is interrupted in places by *Aporias*, where I begin to deconstruct my own deconstruction and (more importantly) offer you the opportunity to write your own sub-text. As I have said, it is a unique and singular deconstructive reading that challenges and encourages you to listen/read/write your own.

Notes

1   Derrida, J. Deconstruction and the other. In R. Kearney (ed) *Dialogues with Contemporary Continental Thinkers: The Phenomenological Heritage*, Manchester: Manchester University Press, 1984, p.124

2   McQuillan, M. Introduction: five strategies for deconstruction. In M.
    McQuillan (ed) *Deconstruction: A Reader*. Edinburgh: Edinburgh
    University Press, 2000, p.4.
3   Ibid p.6
4   Ibid p.5
5   Ibid p.5
6   Ibid p.6
7   Ibid p.6
8   In fact, this is somewhat of an oversimplification, as we will later see.
    However, it will do for now!
9   Barthes R. *The Pleasure of the Text*. New York: Hill and Wang,
    1975, p.67
10 Bennington G. Deconstruction is not what you think, *Art and Design*,
    1988, 4(3/4), pp.6-7.
11 Alan Bass, in the Translator's Introduction to *The Post Card*, notes
    that '*enfant* means "child", from the Latin *infans*, meaning "unable
    to talk"'. Derrida, J. *The Post Card: From Socrates to Freud and
    Beyond*, Chicago: The University of Chicago Press, 1987, p.xx

---

Evidence-Based Medicine:
A New Approach to Teaching
the Practice of Medicine

*Evidence-Based Medicine
Working Group*

A new paradigm for medical practice is emerging. Evidence-based
medicine de-emphasizes intuition,
unsystematic clinical experience,
and pathophysiologic rationale as
sufficient grounds for clinical decision making and stresses the examination of evidence from clinical
research. Evidence-based medicine requires new skills of the physician, including efficient literature

The Annunciation

*And the angel said unto
them, Be not afraid; for
behold, I bring you good
tidings of great joy which
shall be to all the people:
for there is born to you
this day in the city of
David a Saviour, which is
Christ the Lord.* (Luke 2,
10-11)

Introduction
The paper *Evidence-Based
Medicine: a new approach to
teaching the practice of
medicine*[1], published by the
'Evidence-Based Medicine
Working Group' in the pres-

searching and the application of formal rules of evidence evaluating the clinical literature.

An important goal of our medical residency program is to educate physicians in the practice of evidence-based medicine. Strategies include a weekly, formal academic half-day for residents, devoted to learning the necessary skills; recruitment into teaching roles of physicians who practice evidence-based medicine; sharing among faculty of approaches to teaching evidence-based medicine; and providing faculty with feedback on their performance as role models and teachers of evidence-based medicine. The influence of evidence-based medicine on clinical practice and medical education is increasing.

Clinical Scenario

A junior medical resident working in a teaching hospital admits a 43-year-old previously well man who experienced a witnessed grand mal seizure. He had never had a seizure before and had not had any recent head trauma. He drank alcohol once or twice a week and had not had alcohol on the day of the seizure. Findings on physical examination are normal. The patient is given a loading dose of phenytoin intravenously and the drug is continued orally. A computed tomographic head scan is completely normal, and an electroencephalogram shows only nonspecific findings. The patient is very concerned about his risk of

tigious *Journal of the American Medical Association*, presented what amounted to the first manifesto for the self-styled 'new paradigm' of evidence-based medicine (EBM). It is still regularly cited as one of the original sources, and as such, we might expect it to contain a clear, concise and unambiguous exposition of the basic tenets of EBM. As we shall see, however, it is muddled and confusing with no clear structure, and contains a number of contradictions, some of which are quite overt, whilst others become apparent only on a very close reading.

There are a number of possible explanations for why the paper should be so muddled and confusing. First, it might simply be the result of having thirty-one authors. Second, it might be the natural consequence of reporting on new ideas that are not yet fully developed. Third, it might be a more or less deliberate strategy to conceal the fact that the ideas are not fully developed. Fourth, it might be a deliberate strategy to present some radical and potentially unpopular new ideas in a more sympathetic light. And fifth, it might be a combination of some or all of the previous four. My aim in this deconstructive commentary is to un-

seizure recurrence. How might the resident proceed?

The Way of the Past

Faced with this situation as a clinical clerk, the resident was told by her senior resident (who was supported in this view by the attending physician) that the risk of seizure recurrence is high (though he could not put an exact number on it) and that was the information that should be conveyed to the patient. She now follows this path, emphasizing to the patient not to drive, to continue his medication, and to see his family physician in follow-up. The patient leaves in a state of vague trepidation about his risk of subsequent seizure.

The Way of the Future

The resident asks herself whether she knows the prognosis of a first seizure and realizes she does not. She proceeds to the library and, using the Grateful Med program,[1] conducts a computerized literature search. She enters the Medical Subject Headings terms *epilepsy, prognosis,* and *recurrence,* and the program retrieves 25 relevant articles. Surveying the titles, one[2] appears directly relevant. She reviews the paper, finds that it meets criteria she has previously learned for a valid investigation of prognosis,[3] and determines that the results are applicable to her patient. The search costs the resident $2.68, and the entire process (including the trip to the library and the time to make a photocopy of the

cover and explore the confusions and contradictions by examining certain tensions, uncertainties and 'dead ends' in the paper (what Derrida called *aporias*) and more importantly, to speculate on some possible reasons for them.

Aporia

This is, of course, merely one deconstructive reading among many, and as such it carries no authority over and above the paper it is attempting to critique, nor over any other deconstructive reading that you or anyone else might attempt. You might therefore wish to pause at this point and consider what my deconstruction might offer you both as a reader and as a practitioner. In particular, if I am not claiming that my deconstruction is any more 'true' or 'accurate' than the paper I am responding to, then what is the point of a deconstructive reading? This is a question I shall return to later.

Authority and the 'New Paradigm'

The issue of authority is one of a number of tensions which recur throughout the paper. The first thing to note is that the title of the paper, which is often overlooked, advocated EBM not as a new approach to the practice of medicine, but as a new approach to

article) took half an hour.

The results of the relevant study show that the patient risk of recurrence at 1 year is between 43% and 51%, and at 3 years the risk is between 51% and 60%. After a seizure-free period of 18 months his risk of recurrence would likely be less than 20%. She conveys this information to the patient, along with a recommendation that he take his medication, see his family doctor regularly, and have a review of his need for medication if he remains seizure-free for 18 months. The patient leaves with a clear idea of his likely prognosis.

A Paradigm Shift

Thomas Kuhn has described scientific paradigms as ways of looking at the world that define both the problems that can legitimately be addressed and the range of admissible evidence that may bear on their solution.[4] When defects in an existing paradigm accumulate to the extent that the paradigm is no longer tenable, the paradigm is challenged and replaced by a new way of looking at the world. Medical practice is changing, and the change, which involves using the medical literature more effectively in guiding medical practice, is profound enough that it can appropriately be called a paradigm shift.

The foundations of the paradigm shift lie in developments in clinical research over the last 30 years. In 1960, the randomized clinical trial was an oddity. It is now

teaching the practice of medicine. I shall explore the possible reasons for this later, but for now it is sufficient to note that the paper appears to be addressed primarily to senior physicians and academics with a message about how the practice of junior staff could be changed through education. As such, it draws on the existing power hierarchy to promote a 'top down' model of change in which senior physicians act as teachers and role models to junior staff.

Suspicions of a 'top down' approach are reinforced when we consider the authorship of the text. The paper is attributed to the 'Evidence-Based Medicine Working Group' (EBMWG), and lists thirty-one names, including David Sackett, who was later to emerge as the preeminent authority on EBM. Such a marshalling of medical big guns is (at least in part) a statement not only about authorship but also about authority, and implies that although the paper might well contain new and contested material, it is given credibility by sheer weight of numbers. Clearly, however, the paper was not written by thirty-one separate people, and its actual authorship remains unclear, thus providing a certain degree of anonymity against any of its more contentious

accepted that virtually no drug can enter clinical practice without a demonstration of its efficacy in clinical trials. Moreover, the same randomized trial method increasingly is being applied to surgical therapies[5] and diagnostic tests.[6] Meta-analysis is gaining increasing acceptance as a method of summarizing the results of a number of randomized trials, and ultimately may have as profound an effect on setting treatment policy as have randomized trials themselves.[7] While less dramatic, crucial methodological advances have also been made in other areas, such as the assessment of diagnostic tests[8,9] and prognosis.[2]

A new philosophy of medical practice and teaching has followed these methodological advances. This paradigm shift is manifested in a number of ways. A profusion of articles has been published instructing clinicians on how to access,[10] evaluate,[11] and interpret[12] the medical literature. Proposals to apply the principles of clinical epidemiology to day-to-day clinical practice have been put forward.[3] A number of major medical journals have adopted a more informative structured abstract format, which incorporates issues of methods and design into the portion of an article the reader sees first.[13] The American College of Physicians has launched a journal, *ACP Journal Club,* that summarizes new publications of high relevance and methodological rigor.[14] Textbooks that provide a rigorous review of available evi-

statements. The collective authorship therefore serves both to authorise new and controversial ideas and at the same time to 'deauthorise' them; that is, to disguise and conceal their true authorship.

It is here that the nature of the first contradiction or *aporia* in the paper becomes apparent, since this authoritative approach to promoting the new paradigm is in direct contrast to the most basic tenet of EBM, which states that 'the new paradigm puts a much lower value on authority'[2]. On the one hand, then, the authors make every effort to emphasise that EBM challenges existing hierarchies of power which are built on the opinions and authority of senior staff, whereas on the other hand, they are forced to rely on those very structures in order to get their message across.

This contradictory stance, in which medical authority is invoked in order to promote a questioning of that very authority, is again apparent in the very first sentence, which announces to the reader that 'A new paradigm for medical practice is emerging'. This birth announcement sets the scene for the entire paper: it is both authoritative and elusive, and promises at the same time the thrill of innovation and the security of a

dence, including a methods section describing both the methodological criteria used to systematically evaluate the validity of the clinical evidence and the quantitative techniques used for summarizing the evidence, have begun to appear.[15,16] Practice guidelines based on rigorous methodological review of the available evidence are increasingly common.[17] A final manifestation is the growing demand for courses and seminars that instruct physicians on how to make more effective use of the medical literature in their day-to-day patient care.[3]

We call the new paradigm 'evidence-based medicine.'[18] In this article, we describe how this approach differs from prior practice and briefly outline how we are building a residency program in which a key goal is to practice, act as a role model, teach, and help residents become highly adept in evidence-based medicine. We also describe some of the problems educators and medical practitioners face in implementing the new paradigm.

The Former Paradigm

The former paradigm was based on the following assumptions about the knowledge required to guide clinical practice.

1. Unsystematic observations from clinical experience are a valid way of building and maintaining one's knowledge about patient prognosis, the value of diagnostic tests, and the efficacy of treatment.

new order based on a sounder footing than the old. 'A new paradigm ... is emerging', but from where? Are the authors reporting on a wider and already existing trend, or are they referring to their own work? Is the paper in fact self-referential, the first text on/of the new paradigm whose very emergence it is reporting? It is difficult to tell, since the use of the passive case in the above statement successfully serves to conceal its origins.

However, perhaps we do not need to dig too deep in order to understand this ambivalence and elusiveness in presenting the new paradigm. On the one hand, if the authors were to loudly and unambiguously announce the birth of a new (baby) paradigm and claim it as their own (for example: 'we would like to suggest a new paradigm...'), then questions might be raised about whether there actually is a baby; that is, can something so new and tentative really be referred to as a paradigm? (Kuhn, whom the authors invoke to support their claim, would undoubtedly say that it could not). On the other hand, however, if the authors were to make too great a claim that the paradigm is already well-established (for example: 'we would like to explore the new paradigm of EBM...'), then

2. The study and understanding of basic mechanisms of disease and pathophysiologic principles are a sufficient guide for clinical practice.

3. A combination of thorough traditional medical training and common sense is sufficient to allow one to evaluate new tests and treatments.

4. Content expertise and clinical experience are a sufficient base from which to generate valid guidelines for clinical practice.

According to this paradigm clinicians have a number of options for sorting out clinical problems they face. They can reflect on their own clinical experience, reflect on the underlying biology, go to a textbook, or ask a local expert. Reading the introduction and discussion sections of a paper could be considered an appropriate way of gaining the relevant information from a current journal.

This paradigm puts a high value on traditional scientific authority and adherence to standard approaches, and answers are frequently sought from direct contact with local experts or reference to the writings of international experts.[19]

The New Paradigm
The assumptions of the new paradigm are as follows:

1. Clinical experience and the development of clinical instincts (particularly with respect to diagnosis) are a crucial and necessary part of becoming a competent

questions might be raised about the paternity of the baby; in other words, they might be accused of merely building on (adopting) a concept that was conceived by others.

The message suggested by the self-styled label of 'Evidence-Based Medicine Working Group' is that the writers are at the forefront of EBM, and that the 'new paradigm' is indeed being claimed as their own. Their way out of the above dilemma therefore appears to be to cloak the exact moment of the birth in mystery (has it already happened, or is this paper the birth of the paradigm?), whilst obliquely claiming paternity (we are the EBM working group, therefore we gave birth to EBM). If this is so, then the use of the present tense in the sentence 'a new paradigm ... is emerging' is not only disingenuous but dishonest. In a paper that claims to 'put a much lower value on authority', the statement that the work of the group constitutes a new paradigm that *is emerging* offers nothing less than a *fait accomplis*. The group is not *suggesting* a new paradigm, it is not hoping or anticipating that a new paradigm *might* emerge, nor is it reporting on a well-established body of work that is *already accepted* as a new

physician. Many aspects of clinical practice cannot, or will not, ever be adequately tested. Clinical experience and its lessons are particularly important in these situations. At the same time, systematic attempts to record observations in a reproducible and unbiased fashion markedly increase the confidence one can have in knowledge about patient prognosis, the value of diagnostic tests, and the efficacy of treatment. In the absence of systematic observation one must be cautious in the interpretation of information derived from clinical experience and intuition, for it may at times be misleading.

2. The study and understanding of basic mechanisms of disease are necessary but insufficient guides for clinical practice. The rationales for diagnosis and treatment, which follow from basic pathophysiologic principles, may in fact be incorrect, leading to inaccurate predictions about the performance of diagnostic tests and the efficacy of treatments.

3. Understanding certain rules of evidence is necessary to correctly interpret literature on causation, prognosis, diagnostic tests, and treatment strategy.

It follows that clinicians should regularly consult the original literature (and be able to critically appraise the methods and results sections) in solving clinical problems and providing optimal patient care. It also follows that clinicians must be ready to accept and live with uncertainty and to acknow-

paradigm. The new paradigm is emerging whether we like it or not, and the paper in which it is announced is also part of the process and progress of its birth.

Interestingly, this idea that the paper itself is part of the emergence of EBM is borne out towards the end in the first sentence of the 'Conclusion', again written in the passive case, but this time in the perfect tense. Whereas at the start of the paper, a new paradigm *is* emerging, by the end of the paper, 'a new paradigm for medical practice *has arisen*' (my italics). In the space of three thousand words, a new paradigm is born. Furthermore, the only justification we are offered that EBM actually is a new paradigm is based on the authority of thirty-one writers who are jointly making the claim. The group criticises medical interventions which are 'sought from direct contact with local experts or reference to the writings of international experts', and yet nowhere in this paper is there any appeal to external sources of evidence to support the claims of EBM. The tacit message of the opening sentence is that EBM is a new paradigm purely and simply because the EBMWG says that it is.

ledge that management decisions are often made in the face of relative ignorance of their true impact.

The new paradigm puts a much lower value on authority.[20] The underlying belief is that physicians can gain the skills to make independent assessments of evidence and thus evaluate the credibility of opinions being offered by experts. The decreased emphasis on authority does not imply a rejection of what one can learn from colleagues and teachers, whose years of experience have provided them with insight into methods of history taking, physical examination, and diagnostic strategies. This knowledge can never be gained from formal scientific investigation. A final assumption of the new paradigm is that physicians whose practice is based on an understanding of the underlying evidence will provide superior patient care.

Requirements for the Practice of Evidence-based Medicine

The role modeling, practice, and teaching of evidence-based medicine requires skills that are not traditionally part of medical training. These include precisely defining a patient problem, and what information is required to resolve the problem; conducting an efficient search of the literature; selecting the best of the relevant studies and applying rules of evidence to determine their validity[3]; being able to present to col-

Aporia

I have, as yet, not progressed beyond the first sentence of the paper, which proclaimed that 'A new paradigm for medical practice is emerging'. Perhaps this was written as a throwaway line or as a dramatic opening gambit in order to grasp the attention of the reader. Nevertheless, I have taken it at face value, as an example of the writers' true intention insinuating itself into the text when their guard was down. Consequently, I have subjected it to a rather intense 'textual harassment', comparing it to an annunciation, a birth announcement; indeed, to the annunciation, the announcement of a very special and significant birth (you might wish at this point to look again at the quotation at the head of this deconstructive reading).

Before examining the rest of the paper, I would like to raise three issues for you to think about. First, the EBMWG appears to be arguing against authority in a rather authoritarian (or at least, authoritative) tone; they are, in effect, claiming to be the authority on the demise of authority. By devolving authority for clinical decisions down to the level of the individual practi-

leagues in a succinct fashion the content of the article and its strengths and weaknesses; and extracting the clinical message and applying it to the patient problem. We will refer to this process as the critical appraisal exercise.

Evidence-based medicine also involves applying traditional skills of medical training. A sound understanding of pathophysiology is necessary to interpret and apply the results of clinical research. For instance, most patients to whom we would like to generalize the results of randomized trials would, for one reason or another, not have been enrolled in the most relevant study. The patient may be too old, be too sick, have other underlying illnesses, or be uncooperative. Understanding the underlying pathophysiology allows the clinician to better judge whether the results are applicable to the patient at hand and also has a crucial role as a conceptual and memory aid.

Another traditional skill required of the evidence-based physician is a sensitivity to patients' emotional needs. Understanding patients' suffering[21] and how that suffering can be ameliorated by the caring and compassionate physician are fundamental requirements for medical practice. These skills can be acquired through careful observation of patients and of physician role models. Here too, though, the need for systematic study and the limitations of the present evidence must be considered. The new para-

tioner, the EBMWG is also devolving responsibility and accountability, and you might wish to ponder on the irony of a group of authors who are advocating greater individual accountability from behind a collective and largely anonymous title. After all, the paper will be cited and referenced under the name of the working group, and only those readers with access to the original will be able to read the names of the thirty-one authors in small print at the end.

Second, you might wish to consider the wider issue of authority and accountability. If evidence-based practice is concerned with the application of best evidence to practice, and if there are well-defined formal rules for identifying best evidence, then where exactly does accountability lie for your own practice? To use the example given by the EBMWG, if you make a clinical decision based on your own 'unsystematic observations from clinical experience' rather than on the evidence of randomised controlled trials, then you are clearly accountable and responsible for any consequences of your actions. On the other hand, if you override your own experience in favour of the evidence from research, then to what extent is responsibility

digm would call for using the techniques of behavioral science to determine what patients are really looking for from their physicians[22] and how physician and patient behavior affects the outcome of care.[23] Ultimately, randomized trials using different strategies for interacting with patients (such as the randomized trial conducted by Greenfield and colleagues[24] that demonstrated the positive effects of increasing patients' involvement with their care) may be appropriate.

Since evidence-based medicine involves skills of problem defining, searching, evaluating, and applying original medical literature, it is incumbent on residency programs to teach these skills. Understanding the barriers to educating physicians-in-training in evidence-based medicine can lead to more effective teaching strategies.

Evidence-Based Medicine in a Medical Residency

The Internal Medicine Residency Program at McMaster University has an explicit commitment to producing practitioners of evidence-based medicine. While other clinical departments at McMaster have devoted themselves to teaching evidence-based medicine, the commitment is strongest in the Department of Medicine. We will therefore focus on the Internal Medicine Residency in our discussion and briefly outline some of the strategies we are using in imple-

(if not accountability) for your actions shared by the researchers who produced the evidence and, indeed, by the EBMWG for suggesting that you practice in this way?

And third, both the EBMWG paper and this deconstruction are asking you to question traditional sources of authority, although their tones and styles are very different. You might wish to consider the inherent contradictions in each of these approaches. For example, the EBMWG paper seems to be saying, in effect, 'be sceptical of everything (but not of us)', whereas I am saying 'be sceptical of everything (including this message which is telling you to be sceptical)'. This brings to mind the Greek philosopher Eubulides' story of the man from Crete who claimed 'Cretans always lie'. If he is telling the truth, then he is also lying (since it would be true that Cretans always lie). But if he is lying, then he is also telling the truth (since the statement 'Cretans always lie' would be false).

Evidence
As we move on to the second sentence of the paper, the writers begin to outline the nature of EBM, but (in contrast to the opening sentence) in a way that suggests a certain hesita-

menting the paradigm shift.

1. The residents spend each Wednesday afternoon at an academic half-day. At the beginning of each new academic year, the rules of evidence that relate to articles concerning therapy, diagnosis, prognosis, and overviews are reviewed. In subsequent sessions, the discussion is built around a clinical case, and two original articles that bear on the problem are presented. The residents are responsible for critically appraising the articles and arriving at *bottom lines* regarding the strength of evidence and how it bears on the clinical problem. They learn to present the methods and results in a succinct fashion, emphasizing only the key points. A wide-ranging discussion, including issues of underlying pathophysiology and related questions of diagnosis and management, follows presentation of the articles.

The second part of the half-day is devoted to the physical examination. Clinical teachers present optimal techniques of examination with attention to what is known about their reproducibility and accuracy.

2. Facilities for computerized literature searching are available on the teaching medical ward in each of the four teaching hospitals. Costs of searching are absorbed by the residency program. Residents not familiar with computer searching, or the Grateful Med program we use, are instructed at the beginning of the rotation. Research

tion or ambivalence. Thus, they begin by stating what EBM is not: 'Evidence-based medicine de-emphasises intuition, unsystematic clinical experience, and pathophysiologic rationale as sufficient grounds for clinical decision making'. EBM *de-emphasises* these approaches; it takes away their special importance as *sufficient* grounds for decision-making. Something else is required, something more important. Evidence-based medicine therefore 'stresses the examination of evidence from clinical research'. This, in itself, tells us little, except that the physician must take research findings into account in order to obtain a full picture on which to arrive at a clinical decision; hardly sufficient grounds on which to claim a paradigm shift, even back in 1992.

However, if we read further, this is exactly what *is* being suggested:

> Medical practice is changing, and the change, which involves using the medical literature more effectively in guiding medical practice, is profound enough that it can appropriately be called a paradigm shift.

Having argued for a paradigm shift, the writers continue to provide a very cautious and hesitant expo-

in our institution has shown that MEDLINE searching from clinical settings is feasible with brief training.[25] A subsequent investigation demonstrated that internal medicine house staff who have computer access on the ward and feedback concerning their searching do an average of more than 3.6 searches per month.[26] House staff believe that more than 90% of their searches that are stimulated by a patient problem lead to some improvement in patient care.[25]

3. Assessment of searching and critical appraisal skills is being incorporated into the evaluation of residents.

4. We believe that the new paradigm will remain an academic mirage with little relation to the world of day-to-day clinical practice unless physicians-in-training are exposed to role models who practice evidence-based medicine. As a result, the residency program has placed major emphasis on ensuring this exposure.

First, a focus of recruitment for our Department of Medicine faculty has been internists with training in clinical epidemiology. These individuals have the skills and commitment to practice evidence-based medicine. The residency program works to ensure they have clinical teaching roles available to them.

Second, a program of more rigorous evaluation of attending physicians has been instituted. One of the areas evaluated is the extent to which attending physicians are

sition of exactly what that shift entails. Once again, they begin with what it is not: the 'former paradigm' (is it dead already?) was founded on an over-reliance on unsystematic observations, on the study and understanding of disease and pathophysiology, on 'traditional medical training and common sense', and on expertise and experience. They then outline the 'new paradigm', but again in very hesitant (one might almost say negative) terms. Thus the first assumption of the new paradigm is that:

> clinical experience and the development of clinical instincts . . are a crucial and necessary part of becoming a competent physician.

These are the very qualities that were previously *de-emphasised*, and you might be forgiven for not finding very much difference between the old and the new paradigms. However, the rationale for this statement is that 'many aspects of clinical practice cannot, or will not, ever be adequately tested', and so 'Clinical experience and its lessons are particularly important in these situations'.

The second assumption of the new paradigm is that:

effective in teaching evidence-based medicine.

Third, because it is new to both teachers and learners, and because most clinical teachers have observed few role models and have not received formal training, teaching evidence-based medicine is not easy. To help attending physicians improve their skills in this area, we have encouraged them to form partnerships, which involve attending the partner's clinical rounds, making observations, and providing formal feedback. One learns through observation and through criticisms of one's performance. A number of faculty members have participated in this program.

To further facilitate attending physicians' improving their skills, the Department of Medicine held a retreat devoted to sharing strategies for effective clinical teaching. Part of the workshop, attended by more than 30 faculty members, was devoted to teaching evidence-based medicine. Some of the strategies that were adduced are briefly summarized in the next section.

Effective Teaching of Evidence-Based Medicine
Role Modeling
Attending physicians must be enthusiastic, effective role models for the practice of evidence-based medicine (even in high-pressure clinical settings, such as intensive care units). Providing a model goes a long way toward inculcating atti-

The study and understanding of basic mechanisms of disease are necessary but insufficient guides for clinical practice.

Once again, we are told what is insufficient but not what is sufficient for clinical practice. Finally, however, we are offered the third assumption that:

Understanding certain rules of evidence is necessary to correctly interpret literature on causation, prognosis, diagnostic tests, and treatment strategy.

After nearly one thousand words, we are finally told: evidence-based medicine entails 'understanding certain rules of evidence'. Quite what they might be, is at this point still something of a mystery, although it later emerges that they include 'skills of problem-defining, searching, evaluating, and applying original medical literature'.

It gradually becomes apparent that the criteria for evaluating the literature place a high value on randomised controlled trials (RCTs) and meta-analyses, and that there is, in fact, a hierarchy of evidence, although this is never explicitly stated. This is unfortunate, since the reader is left to come to her own conclusions

tudes that lead learners to develop skills in critical appraisal. Acting as a role model involves specifying the strength of evidence that supports clinical decisions. In one case, the teacher can point to a number of large randomized trials, rigorously reviewed and included in a meta-analysis, which allows one to say how many patients one must treat to prevent a death. In other cases, the best evidence may come from accepted practice or one's clinical experience and instincts. The clinical teacher should make it clear to learners on what basis decisions are being made. This can be done efficiently. For instance:

Prospective studies suggest that Mr Jones' risk of a major vascular event in the first year after his infarct is 4%; a meta-analysis of randomized trials of aspirin in this situation suggests a risk reduction of 25%; we would have to treat 100 such patients to prevent an event[27]; given the minimal expense and toxicity of low-dose, enteric-coated aspirin, treating Mr Jones is clearly warranted.

Or:

How long to treat a patient with antibiotics following pneumonia has not been systematically studied; so, my recommendation that we give Mrs Smith 3 days of intravenous antibiotics and treat her for a total of 10 days is arbitrary; somewhat shorter or longer courses of treatment would be equally reasonable.

about how the hierarchy operates. It would appear, from the constant reassurances, that clinical experience and knowledge are rated almost as highly as the findings from RCTs; indeed, that they are essential prerequisites in the judicious application of research evidence. Thus, as we have already seen, 'clinical experience and the development of clinical instincts *are a crucial and necessary part* of becoming a competent physician', and 'the study and understanding of basic mechanisms of disease *are necessary but insufficient guides* for clinical practice' (my italics).

However, a closer reading suggests that this might not be the whole picture. For example, clinical experience is only important in situations where there are no RCTs to support practice, although even then, 'one must be cautious in the interpretation of information derived from clinical experience and intuition, for it may at times be misleading'. Similarly, an understanding of underlying pathophysiology is only important where there is a 'dearth of adequate evidence', suggesting, of course, that such understanding constitutes *inadequate* evidence.

The use of experience and expertise is also seen as

In the latter type of situation, dogmatic or rigid insistence on following a particular course of action would not be appropriate.

Critical Appraisal

It is crucial that critical appraisal issues arise from patient problems that the learner is currently confronting, demonstrating that critical appraisal is a pragmatic and central aspect, not an *academic* or tangential element of optimal patient care. The problem selected for critical appraisal must be one that the learners recognize as important, feel uncertain, and do not fully trust expert opinion; in other words, they must feel it is worth the effort to find out what the literature says on a topic. The likeliest candidate topics are common problems where learners have been exposed to divergent opinions (and thus there is disagreement and/or uncertainty among the learners). The clinical teacher should keep these requirements in mind when considering questions to encourage the learners to address. It can be useful to ask all members of the group their opinion about the clinical problem at hand. One can then ensure that the problem is appropriate for a critical appraisal exercise by asking the group the following questions:

  1. It seems the group is uncertain about the optimal approach. Is that right?

  2. Do you feel it is important for us to sort out this question by going

second best when dealing with the emotional needs of patients. The writers begin with the reassurance that 'another traditional skill required of the evidence-based physician is a sensitivity to patients' emotional needs', such that 'understanding patients' suffering and how that suffering can be ameliorated by the caring and compassionate physician are fundamental requirements for medical practice'. However, even in the case of this 'fundamental requirement' the clinician's judgement is called into question, since 'the new paradigm would call for using the techniques of behavioral science *to determine what patients are really looking for* from their physicians' (my italics). What patients really want in terms of emotional understanding cannot be left to the judgement of the physician, so even when it comes to offering care and compassion, 'ultimately, randomized trials using different strategies for interacting with patients ... may be appropriate'.

What begins to emerge from these examples are two different and contradictory types of hierarchy of evidence. The overt and physician-friendly face of EBM emphasizes, often to the point of distraction,

to the original literature?

Methodological Criteria

Criteria for methodological rigor must be few and simple. Most published criteria can be overwhelming for the novice. Suggested criteria for studies of diagnosis, treatment, and review articles follow:

Diagnosis - Has the diagnostic test been evaluated in a patient sample that included an appropriate spectrum of mild and severe, treated and untreated disease, plus individuals with different but commonly confused disorders? - Was there an independent, blind comparison with a 'gold standard' of diagnosis?[28]

Treatment - Was the assignment of patients to treatments randomized?[29] Were all patients who entered the study accounted for at its conclusion?[29]

Review Articles - Were explicit methods used to determine which articles to include in the review?[30]

As learners become more sophisticated, additional criteria can be introduced. The criteria should not be presented in such a way that fosters nihilism (if the study is not randomized, it is useless and provides no valuable information), but as a way of helping arrive at the strength of inference associated with a clinical decision. Teachers can point out instances in which criteria can be violated without reducing the strength of inference.

how existing skills and expertise continue to be valued. In this scenario, EBM entails the introduction of research-based findings *alongside* the more traditional skills of the physician. There is a hierarchy of evidence, but it is an *inclusive* hierarchy in which clinical experience might carry less weight than the randomised controlled trial, but that the two are somehow used together to produce the 'best evidence' for any clinical problem. The other, less overt and less physician-friendly face of EBM suggests a far more *exclusive* hierarchy in which the findings from RCTs should be applied wherever they exist, and only in cases where there is a 'dearth of adequate evidence', or where certain 'aspects of clinical practice cannot, or will not, ever be adequately tested' should the physician fall back on other forms of evidence.

We can perhaps now begin to see why the writers took such a cautious approach to outlining the sources of evidence for EBM. The underlying and to some extent hidden agenda appears to be to promote the exclusive form of the hierarchy, in which clinical experience, knowledge and expertise should only be applied when there are no RCTs on which to base clinical decisions.

Methods for Scaling the Barriers to the Dissemination of Evidence-Based Medicine
Misapprehensions About Evidence-Based Medicine

In developing the practice and teaching of evidence-based medicine at our institution, we have found that the nature of the new paradigm is sometimes misinterpreted. Recognizing the limitations of intuition, experience, and understanding of pathophysiology in permitting strong inferences may be misinterpreted as rejecting these routes to knowledge. Specific misinterpretations of evidence-based medicine and their corrections follow:

Misinterpretation 1 - Evidence-based medicine ignores clinical experience and clinical intuition.

Correction - On the contrary, it is important to expose learners to exceptional clinicians who have a gift for intuitive diagnosis, a talent for precise observation, and excellent judgment in making difficult management decisions. Untested signs and symptoms should not be rejected out of hand. They may prove extremely useful and ultimately be proved valid through rigorous testing. The more the experienced clinicians can dissect the process they use in diagnosis,[31] and clearly present it to learners, the greater the benefit. Similarly, the gain for students will be greatest when clues to optimal diagnosis and treatment are culled from the barrage of clinical information in a systematic and repro-

However, if stated overtly, such a message would immediately alienate many experienced practitioners. The paper is therefore written in such a way that it is never entirely clear just exactly where clinical experience and expertise fit in the picture of EBM.

Aporia

Having announced the birth of the new paradigm in their opening sentence, the writers then shift down several gears and continue far more cautiously. We are told what EBM is not rather than what it is, what it de-emphasizes rather than what it emphasizes, and the final revelation of what EBM actually is follows almost one thousand words of introductory preamble. Perhaps you would like to consider the significance of such a strategy. My reading is that the eventual message, namely, that EBM is the 'understanding of certain rules of evidence necessary to correctly interpret literature...' is at the same time so banal and so far-reaching that it requires a great deal of disguise.

Its banality lies in its statement of the obvious: the research literature is important and it needs to be correctly interpreted. This is the 'soft' or 'inclusive' form of EBM in which the practitioner uses

ducible fashion.

Institutional experience can also provide important insights. Diagnostic tests may differ in their accuracy depending on the skill of the practitioner. A local expert in, for instance, diagnostic ultrasound may produce far better results than the average from the published literature. The effectiveness and complications associated with therapeutic interventions, particularly surgical procedures, may also differ among institutions. When optimal care is taken to both record observations reproducibly and avoid bias, clinical and institutional experience evolves into the systematic search for knowledge that forms the core of evidence-based medicine.[32]

Misinterpretation 2 - Understanding of basic investigation and pathophysiology plays no part in evidence-based medicine.

Correction - The dearth of adequate evidence demands that clinical problem solving must rely on an understanding of underlying pathophysiology. Moreover, a good understanding of pathophysiology is necessary for interpreting clinical observations and for appropriate interpretation of evidence (especially in deciding on its generalizability).

Misinterpretation 3 - Evidence-based medicine ignores standard aspects of clinical training, such as the physical examination.

Correction - Careful history taking and physical examination provide much, and often the best,

her expertise in order to reach a clinical judgement based on experience, 'clinical instincts' and available research findings. However, in its 'hard' or 'exclusive' form, EBM is revolutionary and potentially alienating. Having claimed that experience and intuition are 'crucial and necessary', the authors later caution us that information derived from these sources might 'at times be misleading', and indeed, that it should only be employed when there is a dearth of evidence from RCTs. In other words, that the clinical experience and expertise of practitioners should be rejected in favour of experience and expertise at reading and interpreting research findings. The writers are therefore walking an extremely thin tightrope: to proclaim something new and revolutionary whilst disguising the true implications of the revolution. We can see, then, that there is as much to be gained in withholding or disguising certain knowledge as there is in presenting it.

Education and Practice
There is yet a further contradiction in the presentation of EBM in this paper. In addition to the question of whether EBM is or is not a new paradigm,

evidence for diagnosis and direct treatment decisions. The clinical teacher of evidence-based medicine must give considerable attention to teaching the methods of history taking and clinical examination, with particular attention to which items have demonstrated validity and to strategies that enhance observer agreement.

Barriers to Teaching Evidence-Based Medicine

Difficulties we have encountered in teaching evidence-based medicine include the following:

1. Many house staff start with rudimentary critical appraisal skills and the topic may be threatening for them.

2. People like quick and easy answers. Cookbook medicine has its appeal. Critical appraisal involves additional time and effort and may be perceived as inefficient and distracting from the real goal (to provide optimal care for patients).

3. For many clinical questions, high quality evidence is lacking. If such questions predominate in attempts to introduce critical appraisal, a sense of futility can result.

4. The concepts of evidence-based medicine are met with skepticism by many faculty members who are therefore unenthusiastic about modifying their teaching and practice in accordance with its dictates.

These problems can be ameliorated by the use of the strategies

and on what grounds such a claim could rightfully be made, it is unclear just what it is that is claimed to be new. The announcement, the annunciation, is that 'A new paradigm for medical practice is emerging'. Why, then, does the title of the paper proclaim 'a new approach to *teaching* the practice of medicine' rather than a new approach to practice *per se*? Certainly, much of the paper is concerned with education rather than directly with medicine, and whereas the term 'evidence based medicine' is most often used to denote a new approach to practice, the emphasis on education is invoked at key moments throughout the text. The question we might ask ourselves, then, is why the writers should take such a confusing stance that shifts uneasily between two aspects of EBM without ever fully resolving the issue. There are a number of possible answers to this question.

First, whilst EBM would appear to have a predominantly practice-based agenda, most of the writers are employed as academics and educationalists whose main influence on practice is through educating and supervising others. In introducing a new paradigm for practice, they leave themselves open not only to the usual charge of being theorists who do not under-

described in the previous section on effective teaching of evidence-based medicine. Threat can be reduced by making a contract with the residents, which sets out modest and achievable goals, and further reduced by the attending physician role modeling the practice of evidence-based medicine. Inefficiency can be reduced by teaching effective searching skills and simple guidelines for assessing the validity of the papers. In addition, one can emphasize that critical appraisal as a strategy for solving clinical problems is most appropriate when the problems are common in one's own practice. Futility can be reduced by, particularly initially, targeting critical appraisal exercises to areas in which there is likely to be high-quality evidence that will affect clinical decisions. Skepticism of faculty members can be reduced by the availability of 'quick and dirty' (as well as more sophisticated) courses on critical appraisal of evidence and by the teaching partnerships and teaching workshops described earlier.

Many problems in the practice and teaching of evidence-based medicine remain. Many physicians, including both residents and faculty members, are still skeptical about the tenets of the new paradigm. A medical residency is full of competing demands, and the appropriate balance between goals is not always evident. At the same time, we are buoyed by the number of residents and faculty who have

stand the 'real world' of medical practice, but also to their own critique of being the very 'experts' that evidence-based practitioners are being urged to avoid. If these academics are to establish themselves as credible authorities on medical practice and the instigators of a new paradigm, then it is important that EBM has a firm foundation in their own sphere of authority; that is, in education.

Second, one of the stated aims of the paper is to promote the educational programme at McMasters University, which 'has an explicit commitment to producing practitioners of evidence-based medicine'. By associating EBM with 'a new approach to teaching the practice of medicine', the writers are sending out a strong message that the best way of taking part in the 'paradigm shift' to EBM is through enrolling on a course at McMasters University. Indeed, a large section of the paper is devoted to describing the Internal Medicine Residency Program in what amounts to little more than a prospectus and advertisement for the course. The educational link therefore has clear financial implications for both the university (extra course fees) and the individuals on the EBMWG (lucrative consultancy fees).

On this reading, then,

enthusiastically adopted the new approach and found ways to integrate it into their learning and practice.

Barriers to Practising Evidence-Based Medicine

Even if our residency program is successful in producing graduates who enter the world of clinical practice enthusiastic to apply what they have learned about evidence-based medicine, they will face difficult challenges. Economic constraints and counterproductive incentives may compete with the dictates of evidence as determinants of clinical decisions; the relevant literature may not be readily accessible; and the time available may be insufficient to carefully review the evidence (which may be voluminous) relevant to a pressing clinical problem.

Some solutions to these problems are already available. Optimal integration of computer technology into clinical practice facilitates finding and accessing evidence. Reference to literature overviews meeting scientific principles[30,33] and collections of methodologically sound and highly relevant articles[14] can markedly increase efficiency. Other solutions will emerge over time. Health educators will continue to find better ways of role modeling and teaching evidence-based medicine. Standards in writing reviews and texts are likely to change, with a greater focus on methodological rigor.[15,16] Evidence-based summar-

the paradigm shift is motivated not only (as the writers claim) by changes in medical practice, but (as with most paradigm shifts) by considerations of power and economics. There is, however, a third reason for the educational emphasis on EBM, which concerns the evidence for the new paradigm. If EBM tells us that all practice is to be based on research evidence, then it is reasonable to ask what the evidence is to support the practice of EBM. Interestingly, the question of what is the evidence for EBM is not framed by the writers in this way, but rather as 'Does *teaching and learning* evidence-based medicine improve patient outcomes?' (my italics). On first reading, this would appear to be the wrong question. Surely we should be interested in whether the *practice* of EBM improves patient outcomes. However, I have already discussed some of the reasons why the writers might wish to associate patient outcomes with education rather than directly with practice (money and power!), and another reason becomes apparent as we read a little further:

> The proof of the pudding of evidence-based medicine lies in whether patients cared for in this fashion enjoy better

ies will therefore become increasingly available. Practical approaches to making evidence-based summaries easier to apply in clinical practice, many based on computer technology, will be developed and expanded. As described earlier, we are already using computer searching on the ward. In the future, the results of diagnostic tests may be provided with the associated sensitivity, specificity, and likelihood ratios. Health policymakers may find that the structure of medical practice must be shifted in basic ways to facilitate the practice of evidence-based medicine. Increasingly, scientific overviews will be systematically integrated with information regarding toxicity and side effects, cost, and the consequences of alternative courses of action to develop clinical policy guidelines.[34] The prospects for these developments are both bright and exciting.

Does Teaching and Learning Evidence-Based Medicine Improve Patient Outcomes?

The proof of the pudding of evidence-based medicine lies in whether patients cared for in this fashion enjoy better health. This proof is no more achievable for the new paradigm than it is for the old, for no long-term randomized trials of traditional and evidence-based medical education are likely to be carried out. What we do have are a number of short-term studies which confirm that the skills of evidence-based medicine can be taught to

health. This proof is no more achievable for the new paradigm than it is for the old, for no long-term randomized trials of traditional and evidence-based medical education are likely to be carried out.

On first sight, the writers appear to have rejected their own new paradigm, since there are no long-term RCTs to support either the practice or the teaching of EBM. However, whilst suitable evidence to support the *practice* of EBM is unlikely to be forthcoming in the near future, there were, at the time of writing their paper, 'a number of short-term studies which confirm that the skills of evidence-based medicine can be taught to medical students and medical residents'. Perhaps, but that does not, of course, imply that those students will use their new skills, nor that those skills equate with better practice. In addition to these short-term studies, there was also a study which 'compared the graduates of a medical school that operates under the new paradigm with the graduates of a traditional school', which 'suggest[s] that the teaching of evidence-based medicine may help graduates stay up-to-date'. In fact, this latter study demonstrated merely that McMasters

medical students[35] and medical residents.[36] In addition, a study compared the graduates of a medical school that operates under the new paradigm (McMaster) with the graduates of a traditional school. A random sample of McMaster graduates who had chosen careers in family medicine were more knowledgeable with respect to current therapeutic guidelines in the treatment of hypertension than were the graduates of the traditional school.[37] These results suggest that the teaching of evidence-based medicine may help graduates stay up-to-date. Further evaluation of the evidence-based medicine approach is necessary.

Our advocating evidence-based medicine in the absence of definitive evidence of its superiority in improving patient outcomes may appear to be an internal contradiction. As has been pointed out, however, evidence-based medicine does not advocate a rejection of all innovations in the absence of definitive evidence. When definitive evidence is not available, one must fall back on weaker evidence (such as the comparison of graduates of two medical schools that use different approaches cited above) and on biologic rationale. The rationale in this case is that physicians who are up-to-date as a function of their ability to read the current literature critically, and are able to distinguish strong from weaker evidence, are likely to be more judicious in the therapy they recommend. Physi-

graduates 'were more knowledgeable with respect to current therapeutic guidelines in the treatment of hypertension than were graduates of the traditional school', which hardly constitutes sound evidence for the claim that the new paradigm of EBM leads to better outcomes for patients than the old paradigm.

Aporia

It is notable that the confused and distorted messages being promoted in the paper extend to the very nature of EBM itself. In particular, it is never fully made clear whether EBM is being proposed as a new paradigm of practice or a new paradigm of education. As you have seen, my reading is that whereas it suits the writers to proclaim that 'A new paradigm for medical practice is emerging', such a paradigm can only be defended from critique as a 'new approach to teaching the practice of medicine'. Furthermore, a new approach to practice is firmly in the public domain whereas a new teaching method is under the academic and financial control of the institution and the individuals who developed it. The EBMWG might well denounce the authority and credibility of experts in medicine, but they are quick to proclaim their own

cians who understand the properties of diagnostic tests and are able to use a quantitative approach to those tests are likely to make more accurate diagnoses. While this rationale appears compelling to us, compelling rationale has often proved misleading. Until more definitive evidence is adduced, adoption of evidence-based medicine should appropriately be restricted to two groups. One group comprises those who find the rationale compelling, and thus believe that use of the evidence-based medicine approach is likely to improve clinical care. A second group comprises those who, while skeptical of improvements in patient outcome, believe it is very unlikely that deterioration in care results from the evidence-based approach and who find that the practice of medicine in the new paradigm is more exciting and fun.

Conclusion

Based on an awareness of the limitations of traditional determinants of clinical decisions, a new paradigm for medical practice has arisen. Evidence-based medicine deals directly with the uncertainties of clinical medicine and has the potential for transforming the education and practice of the next generation of physicians. These physicians will continue to face an exploding volume of literature, rapid introduction of new technologies, deepening concern about burgeoning medical costs, and increasing attention to the

authority and credibility as experts in the teaching of medicine.

The Evidence for Evidence-Based Medicine

Not surprisingly, however, the almost total lack of evidence to support EBM does *not* lead the writers to reject it as failing to satisfy its own criteria. However, their denial of its shortcomings can only serve to produce yet another site of conflict and tension. The writers begin their defence of EBM by attempting to play down the lack of evidence to support it. Thus, in the absence of 'definitive evidence', it is permissible to fall back on 'weaker evidence' and biologic rationale. In this case, however, the evidence is not only weak (in the writers' sense of not deriving from a RCT), but is largely irrelevant, since it establishes no links whatsoever (either causal or associative) between the practice of EBM and improved patient care.

The writers therefore attempt two rather circuitous 'biologic rationales' for EBM. Firstly, they argue that physicians who are up to date with the current literature through being able to read it critically (one of the basic tenets of EBM) are likely to be more judicious in the therapy they recommend

quality and outcomes of medical care. The likelihood that evidence-based medicine can help ameliorate these problems should encourage its dissemination.

Evidence-based medicine will require new skills for the physician, skills that residency programs should be equipped to teach. While strategies for inculcating the principles of evidence-based medicine remain to be refined, initial experience has revealed a number of effective approaches. Incorporating these practices into postgraduate medical education and continuing to work on their further development will result in more rapid dissemination and integration of the new paradigm into medical practice.

The Evidence-Based Medicine Working Group comprised the following: Gordon Guyatt (chair), MD, MSc, John Cairns, MD, David Churchill, MD, MSc, Deborah Cook, MD, MSc, Brian Haynes, MD, MSc, PhD, Jack Hirsh, MD, Jan Irvine, MD, MSc, Mark Levine, MD, MSc, Mitchell Levine, MD, MSc, Jim Nishikawa, MD, and David Sackett, MD, MSc, Departments of Medicine and Clinical Epidemiology and Biostatistics, McMaster University, Hamilton, Ontario; Patrick Brill-Edwards, MD, Hertzel Gerstein, MD, MSc, Jim Gibson, MD, Roman Jaeschke, MD, MSc, Anthony Kerigan, MD, MSc, Alan Neville, MD, and Akbar Panju, MD, Department of Medicine, McMaster University; Allan Detsky, MD, PhD, Department of Clinical Epidemiology and Biostatistics, McMaster University and Departments of Health Administration and Medicine, University of Toronto (Ontario); Murray

simply because they are reading the literature critically. This, of course is a circular argument, since they are attempting to justify the tenets of EBM by appealing to those very tenets, rather like claiming that RCTs are the gold standard of research because the trials are controlled and randomised. Secondly, they argue that physicians who understand the properties of diagnostic tests are likely to make more accurate diagnoses. This might, of course, appear to be a statement of the obvious, although elsewhere they point out that 'the rationales for diagnosis and treatment ... may in fact be incorrect, leading to inaccurate predictions about the performance of diagnostic tests and the efficacy of treatments'. Indeed, one of the tenets of EBM is to distrust such 'common sense' rationale, and the writers are eventually forced to accept this very point, and note that 'while this rationale appears compelling to us, compelling rationale has often proved misleading'. Ultimately, then, EBM fails to satisfy its own criterion that all practice (including the practice of EBM) should be based on sound evidence.

However, the writers remain undeterred, since 'evidence-based medicine

Enkin, MD, Departments of Clinical Epidemiology and Biostatistics and Obstetrics and Gynaecology, McMaster University; Pamela Frid, MD, Department of Pediatrics, Queen's University, Kingston, Ontario; Martha Gerrity, MD, Department of Medicine, University of North Carolina, Chapel Hill; Andreas Laupacis, MD, MSc, Department of Clinical Epidemiology and Biostatistics, McMaster University and Department of Medicine, University of Ottawa (Ontario); Valerie Lawrence, MD, Department of Medicine, University of Texas Health Science Center at San Antonio and Andie L. Murphy Memorial Veterans Hospital, San Antonio, Tex; Joel Menard MD, Centre de Médicine Trezentize Cardio-Vasculaires, Paris, France; Virginia Moyer, MD, Department of Pediatrics, University of Texas, Houston; Cynthia Mulrow, MD, Department of Medicine, University of Texas, San Antonio; Paul Links, MD, MSc, Department of Psychiatry, McMaster University; Andrew Oxman, MD, MSc, Departments of Clinical Epidemiology and Biostatistics and Family Medicine, McMaster University; Jack Sinclair, MD, Departments of Clinical Epidemiology and Biostatistics and Pediatrics, McMaster University; and Peter Tugwell, MD, MSc, Department of Medicine, University of Ottawa (Ontario).

Drs Cook and Guyatt are Career Scientists of the Ontario Ministry of Health. Dr Haynes is a National Health Scientist, National Health Research and Development Program, Canada. Drs Jaeschke and Cook are Scholars of the St Joseph's Hospital Foundation, Hamilton, Ontario.

References

1   Lindberg DA. Information systems to support medical practice and scientific

does not advocate a rejection of all innovations in the absence of definitive evidence'. This is subtly different from the claim they make elsewhere that 'many aspects of clinical practice cannot, or will not, ever be adequately tested'. It is one thing to have to 'accept and live with uncertainty' with regard to established treatment interventions that are as yet untested, but would advocates of EBM really condone the introduction of, for example, an innovative new drug that had not undergone an RCT? Clearly not, since the writers claim elsewhere that 'it is now accepted that virtually no drug can enter clinical practice without a demonstration of its efficacy in clinical trials'. And yet that is exactly what the writers are advocating for EBM itself, in one of the most revealing and yet least quoted paragraphs of the entire paper. Having previously admitted that the proof of whether EBM leads to better patient care 'is no more achievable for the new paradigm than it is for the old, for no long-term randomised trials of traditional and evidence-based medical education are likely to be carried out', they then give the remarkable advice to would-be evidence-based physicians that:

discovery. *Methods Inform Med.*
1989; 28:202-206.

2   Hart YM, Sander JW, Johnson AL,
Shorvon SD. National general
practice study of epilepsy:
recurrence after a first seizure.
Lancet. 1990; 336:1271-1274.

3   Sackett DL, Haynes RB, Guyatt
GH, Tugwell P. *Clinical Epidemi-
ology: A Basic Science for
Clinical Medicine.* 2nd ed.
Boston, Mass: Little Brown & Co
Inc; 1991: 173-186.

4   Kuhn TS. *The Structure of
Scientific Revolutions.* Chicago,
Ill: University of Chicago Press;
1970.

5   European Carotid Surgery
Trialists' Collaborative Group.
MEC European Carotid Surgery
Trial: interim results for symptom-
atic patients with severe (70-
99%) or with mild (0-29%)
carotid stenosis. *Lancet.* 1991;
337:1235-I243.

6   Larsen ML, Horder M, Mogensen
EF. Effect of long-term monitoring of glycosylated hemoglobin
levels in insulin dependent
diabetes mellitus. *N Engl J Med.*
1990; 323:1021-1025.

7   L'Abbe KA, Detsky AS, O'Rourke
K. Meta-analysis in clinical
research. *Ann Intern Med.* 1987;
107:224-233.

8   Ransohoff DF, Feinstein AR.
Problems of spectrum and bias
in evaluating the efficacy of
diagnostic tests. *N Engl J Med.*
1978; 299:926-930.

9   Nierenberg AA, Feinstein AR.
How to evaluate a diagnostic
market test: lessons from the rise

Until more definitive
evidence is adduced
[which, as they say
above, is unlikely] adop-
tion of evidence-based
medicine should appropri-
ately be restricted to
two groups. One group
comprises those who find
the rationale compelling
[they are referring to
the two 'biologic ration-
ales discussed above],
and thus believe that use
of the evidence-based
medicine approach is
likely to improve clini-
cal care. A second group
comprises those who,
while skeptical of
improvements in patient
outcome, believe it is
very unlikely that deter-
ioration in care results
from the evidence-based
approach and who find
that the practice of
medicine in the new para-
digm is more exciting and
fun.

Aporia

*We have now reached the
most fundamental schism or
aporia in the entire argument for EBM as it was
propounded by the working
group; that it fails utterly to meet its own criteria
for acceptance as a new
form of practice. I suggest
that you now re-read the
previous quotation, this
time substituting the words
'new drug treatment' or
'new surgical procedure'
for 'evidence-based*

and fall of dexamethasone suppression test. *JAMA.* 1988; 259:1699-1702.

10 Haynes RB, McKibbon KA, Fitzgerald D, Guyatt GH, Walker CJ, Sackett DL. How to keep up with the medical literature, V: access by personal computer to the medical literature. *Ann Intern Med.* 1986; 105:810-816.

11 Bulpitt CJ. Confidence intervals. *Lancet.* 1987; 1:494-497.

12 Godfrey K. Simple linear regression in medical research. *N Engl J Med.* 1985; 313:1629-I636.

13 Haynes RB, Mulrow CD, Huth EU, Altman DG, Gardner MJ. More informative abstracts revisited. *Ann Intern Med.* 1990; 113:69-76.

14 Haynes RB. The origins and aspirations of ACP Journal Club. *Ann Intern Med.* 1991; 114 (*ACP J Club.* suppl 1):A18.

15 Chalmers I, Enklin M, Keirse MJNC, eds. *Effective Care in Pregnancy and Childbirth.* New York, NY: Oxford University Press Inc; 1989.

16 Sinclair JC, Braken MB, eds. *Effective Care of the Newborn Infant.* New York, NY: Oxford University Press Inc; 1992.

17 Audet AM, Greenfield S, Field M. Medical practice guidelines: current activities and future directions. *Ann Intern Med.* 1990; 113:709-714.

18 Guyatt GH. Evidence-based medicine. *Ann Intern Med.* 1991; 114 (*ACP J Club.* suppl 2):A-16.

19 Light DW. Uncertainty and

practice'. Is the EBMWG really suggesting that (for example) a new and untested surgical procedure should be adopted by practitioners who 'while skeptical of improvements in patient outcomes, believe it is very unlikely that deterioration in care results from [it] and who find that [it] is more exciting and fun'? Ultimately, the message that this paper is promoting is that all practice should be based on sound evidence, preferably from RCTs, except the practice of EBM, which should be based rather on the amount of excitement and fun that it generates in the practitioner. Not surprisingly, this passage of the paper is never cited by the advocates of EBM.

Conclusion
We have seen, then, that the paper which introduced the self-styled 'new paradigm' of evidence-based practice to the discipline of medicine was full of ambiguity, evasion and contradiction. For me, the key to understanding this paper and the curious style in which it was written lies in the authors' invocation of Thomas Kuhn and the idea of a paradigm shift. Judged according to Kuhn's criteria, the annunciation that 'a new paradigm is emerging' is clearly premature; at the time of

control in professional training. *J Health Soc Behav.* 1979; 20:310-322.

20 Chalmers I. Scientific inquiry and authoritarianism in perinatal care and education. *Birth.* 1983; 10:151-164.

21 Cassell EJ. The nature of suffering and the goals of medicine. *N Engl J Med.* 1982; 306:639-645.

22 Ende J, Kazis L, Ash A, Moskowitz MA. Measuring patients' desire for autonomy: decision-making and information-seeking preferences among medical patients. *J Gen Intern Med.* 1989; 4:23-30.

23 Carter WB, Inui TS, Kulkull WA, Haigh VH. Outcome-based doctor-patient interaction analysis. *Med Care.* 1982; 20:550-556.

24 Greenfield S, Kaplan S, Ware JE Jr. Expanding patient involvement in care: effects on patient outcomes. *Ann Intern Med.* 1985; 102:520-528.

25 Haynes RB, McKibbon A, Walker CJ, Ryan N, Fitzgerald D, Ramsden ME. Online access to MEDLINE in clinical settings: a study of use and usefulness. *Ann Intern Med.* 1990; 112:78-84.

26 McKibbon KA, Haynes RB, Johnston ME, Walker CJ. A study to enhance clinical end-user MEDLINE search skills: design and baseline findings. In: Clayton PD, ed. *Proceedings of the Fifth Annual Symposium on Computer Applications in Medical Care, November 1991;*

publication in 1992, EBM did not constitute a new paradigm, although the extent to which the prophesy of a new paradigm was self-fulfilling is open to debate. But, as Kuhn pointed out, paradigm shifts are always precursors to power shifts, and by establishing themselves as the founders of a new paradigm, the authors could be seen to be making a bid for the power to determine how the teaching and practice of medicine might develop.

However, the paradigm clearly must be accepted not only by academics but by the practitioners who constitute the vast majority of the membership of the discipline. Seen in this light, then, the aim of the paper was not to provide a clear explication of EBM, which might well prove too challenging and even distasteful to practitioners in its rejection of their experience and expertise. Rather, the aim was to establish the authors as dominant figures, indeed as the leaders of the new paradigm whilst at the same time obscuring the contradictions which lie in the finer details. If this is so, then the aim of the authors in writing this paper was not to advance knowledge but to seize power. It was only four years later, once EBM was firmly established, that

Washington, DC. New York, NY: McGraw-Hill International Book Co; 1992: 73-77.

27 Laupacis A, Sackett DL, Roberts RS. An assessment of clinically useful measures of the consequences of treatment. *N Engl J. Med.* 1988; 318:1728-1733.

28 Department of Clinical Epidemiology and Biostatistics, McMaster University. How to read clinical journals, II: to learn about a diagnostic test. *Can Med Assoc J.* 198I; 124:703-710.

29 Department of Clinical Epidemiology and Biostatistics, McMaster University. How to read clinical journals, V: to distinguish useful from useless or even harmful therapy. *Can Med Assoc J.* 1981; 124:1156-1162.

30 Oxman AD, Guyatt GH. Guidelines for reading literature reviews. *Can Med Assoc J.* 1983; 138:697-703.

31 Campbell EJM. The diagnosing mind. *Lancet* 1987; I:849-85I.

32 Feinstein AR. What kind of basic science for clinical medicine? *N Engl J. Med.* 1970; 283:847-853.

33 Mulrow CD. The medical review article: state of the science. *Ann intern Med.* 1987; 106:485-488.

34 Eddy DM. Guidelines for policy statements: the explicit approach. *JAMA.* I990, 263:2239-2243.

35 Bennett KJ, Sackett DL, Haynes RB, et al. A controlled trial of teaching critical appraisal of the clinical literature to medical

Sackett revealed that, in his view, individual clinical expertise should play only a very limited role in medicine, and that 'the randomised trial, and especially the systematic review of several randomised trials ... has become the "gold standard" for judging whether a treatment does more good than harm'[3]. How different this statement is from his earlier criterion for adopting EBM itself, namely that it should be 'more exciting and fun'.

Aporia
You have probably been undertaking your own deconstructive reading of the EBMWG paper (however informally) as you read my text. At this point, you might also like to deconstruct my deconstruction of EBM, and in particular, to consider:

- *What was my agenda in deconstructing this paper? Was I concerned to enhance my knowledge, my power, or something else?*
- *To what extent have I 'read in' my own biases and preconceptions?*
- *Why have I devoted so much time and energy to deconstructing the opening sentence? Why did this hold so much significance for me?*
- *What was the significance for me of the quotation at the head of this chapter? What does it say*

students. *JAMA.* 1987;
257:2451-2454.

36 Kitchens JM, Pfeifer MP.
Teaching residents to read the
medical literature: a controlled
trial of a curriculum in critical
appraisal/clinical epidemiology.
J Gen Intern Med. 1989; 4:384-
387.

37 Shin J, Haynes RB. Does a
problem-based, self directed
undergraduate medical
curriculum promote continuing
clinical competence? *Clin Res.*
1991; 39:143A.

*about the way I view the
EBMWG and their paper?*

Notes

1 Evidence-Based Medicine
   Working Group. Evidence-
   based medicine: a new
   approach to teaching the
   practice of medicine,
   JAMA. 1992; 268:2420-
   2425.

2 Unless otherwise stated,
   all quotations are from
   Evidence-Based Medicine
   Working Group, *op. cit.*

3 Sackett DL, Rosenberg
   WMC, Gray JAM, Haynes RB
   & Richardson WS. Evidence
   based medicine: what it
   is and what it isn't.
   BJM. 1996; 312:71-72.

Deconstruction 2

That dangerous supplement...

Through this sequence of supplements a necessity is announced: that of an infinite chain, ineluctably multiplying the supplementary mediations that produce the sense of the very thing they defer: the mirage of the thing itself, of immediate presence, of ordinary perception.[1]

Here, then, is the scenario. R is invited by a journal editor to write a paper on 'diversity'[2]. He asks F to collaborate on a deconstruction of the way that the concept is employed in nursing. However, R becomes rather carried away by the writing process and produces a more or less complete paper, which he sends to F for additions. F finds it difficult to prise open the text, and instead adds a number of substantial annotations. R is in a quandary: having invited F to collaborate, he is now unsure how to incorporate her extensive notes into the body of the text. This is not only a question of structure, but also one of content, since F's contribution would significantly broaden the focus of R's original paper. Besides, the text is already approaching the word limit set by the journal. R experiences a certain panic.

But there is yet another problem. R's paper warns of the seduction of assimilation, of becoming a part of something bigger, and thereby submitting oneself to rules/structures/language games that are not one's own. R called instead for a stance of *différance*, of toleration and acceptance of epistemological, ontological, and indeed, logical inconsistencies, of an indefinite deferral of judgement. What, then, of F's annotations? Should they not *supplement* R's paper rather than being subsumed/consumed by it?

Derrida had something to say on the question of supplements. His book *Of Grammatology*[3] is a 350-page deconstruction of the 'Spoken word:written word' duality, in which he textually harasses a range of writers from Plato to Lévi-Strauss for placing speech above writing, for considering writing as a supplement to speech. Much of the book is taken up with a deconstruction of Rousseau, and in particular, of his books *Emile* and *Confessions*. At the heart of Rousseau's writing is a dichotomy between the natural and the artificial, which is articulated as the 'Nature: culture' polarity. For Rousseau, culture is a corrupting force that upsets the natural balance of society and of the world, hence the necessity for Emile to be educated in the forest away from the influence of civilisation. Similarly, Rousseau saw writing as a corrupting force that originally led to 'the degeneracy of culture and the disruption of the community'[4] by removing the necessity for face-to-face human contact. Writing is dangerous, 'it is a violence done to the natural destiny of speech'[5]. As Derrida points out, for Rousseau:

> Languages are made to be spoken, writing serves only as a supplement to speech.... Speech represents thought by conventional signs, and writing represents the same with regard to speech. Thus the art of writing is nothing but a mediated representation of thought.[6]

Writing, then, is a dangerous supplement to speech. Unfortunately, it is also a necessary supplement; indeed, Rousseau made his name and his living from the written word.

Derrida's deconstruction of this position focusses on 'that dangerous supplement', and the way in which the French word *suppléer* has two meanings 'whose cohabitation is as strange as it is necessary'[7]. Firstly, it means to add *to*, as in the sense of a food supplement that enhances one's diet. Thus, 'the supplement adds itself, it is a surplus, a plenitude enriching another plenitude, the *fullest measure* of presence'[8]. But it also means a substitute *for*, in the way that a food supplement can *totally replace* food itself. Thus, 'the supplement supplements. It adds only to replace. It intervenes or insinuates itself in-the-place-of; if it fills, it is as if one fills a void'[9]. As we shall see later, one of Derrida's key strategies of deconstruction is to identify words such as *suppléer* that have a double meaning or (as he says) 'two significations' (and which he compared elsewhere to the levers of railway points, 'the delicate levers which pass between the legs of a word and itself'[10]), and to show how they might deliberately or inadvertently send the text off in a new direction.

Derrida points out that, for Rousseau, writing is seen as a dangerous and destructive *addition* to the perfect state of being that is face-to-face spoken communication. But it is also a *necessary* supplement (not least because Rousseau earned his living from it), and so spoken communication clearly does *not* represent a perfect state. Furthermore, Rousseau is employing both meanings of 'supplement' indiscriminately and interchangeably:

> We shall constantly have to confirm that both operate within Rousseau's texts. But the inflexion varies from moment to moment. Each of the two significations is by turns effaced or becomes discretely vague in the presence of the other.[11]

Rousseau's key argument is based around a 'Nature:culture', 'Speaking: writing' polarity, in which the first term is naturally good but becomes corrupted by the addition of (a supplement *to*) the second. However, Derrida breaks down the polarity of opposites by showing how the second term is implicit in, and can stand in for (a supplement *for*) the first. Writing is, at the same time, the polar opposite of speech and also an essential addition to it. Rousseau's texts thus deconstruct themselves. Rousseau also uses the term 'dangerous supplement' to refer to a

> condition almost unintelligible and inconceivable ... which cheats nature and saves up for young men of my temperament many forms of excess at the expense of their health, strength, and, sometimes, their life.[12]

Just as writing is supplementary to speech, so the 'unintelligible and inconceivable' practice of masturbation is supplementary to sexual intercourse. As Rousseau continued, 'I had observed that intercourse with women distinctly aggravated my ill-health. The corresponding vice [of masturbation], of which I have never been able to cure myself completely, appeared to me to produce less injurious results'[13]. Derrida pointed out that, for Rousseau, just as masturbation supplemented (added to, replaced) 'intercourse with women', so women (and, in particular, his mistress Thérèse) supplemented (added to, replaced) his foster mother 'mamma', who in turn supplemented (added to, replaced) his biological mother who died giving birth to him, and who, for Derrida, 'was also in a certain way a supplement from the first trace....'[14] Here is

the chain of supplements'[15]. Thus:

> Through this sequence of supplements a necessity is announced: that
> of an infinite chain, ineluctably multiplying the supplementary media-
> tions that produce the sense of the very thing they defer; the mirage of
> the thing itself, of immediate presence, of originary perception.[16]

And so back to writing (which, in common with masturbation, is traditionally accomplished with the right hand and a vivid imagination).

The 'infinite chain', the 'mirage of the thing itself' and the 'multiplying
[of] the supplementary mediations' suggest 'the absence of the referent
or the transcendental signified. *There is nothing outside of the text*'[17].
Every reading of a text produces a new text, and every reading of that
new text produces still further texts in 'the fall into the abyss of
deconstruction.... Thus a further deconstruction deconstructs
deconstruction, both as the search for a foundation, and as the pleasure
of the bottomless'[18]. Deconstruction, like masturbation, is a dangerous
supplement, both a corrupting addition and a necessity to the text itself.

Below, then, is a thesis (con-text) in the left-hand column that began
its life as a deconstructive reading (sub-text/supplement), and a further
deconstructive reading (sub-sub-text/supplement) of that thesis in the
right hand column. This is followed by two critiques[19] of R's paper after it
was published in *Nurse Education Today*, along with R's response to
those critiques[20]. All three latter papers were published together in a
subsequent edition of *Nurse Education Today*. Although these papers are
not, technically speaking, deconstructions, they effectively illustrate the
point that the number of supplements generated by any paper is
potentially infinite.

Notes

1   Derrida, J. *Of Grammatology*, Baltimore: The Johns Hopkins
     University Press, 1976, p.157
2   Rolfe, G. Faking a difference: evidence-based nursing and the
     illusion of diversity, *Nurse Education Today*, 2002, 22, pp.3-12
3   Derrida, op. cit.
4   Ibid., p.144
5   Ibid., p.144

6   Rousseau, cited in ibid., p.144

7   Ibid., p.144

8   Ibid., p.144, Derrida's emphasis

9   Ibid., p.145

10 Derrida, J. (1980) *The Postcard*, Chicago: University of Chicago
    Press, p.78

11 Derrida, op. cit., p.145

12 Rousseau, cited in ibid., p.149

13 Ibid., p.156

14 Derrida uses the term 'trace' to refer to the 'memory', the 'remains'
    of an ideal state that never actually occurred. In this case, the 'first
    trace' is Rousseau's (our) 'memory' of the ideal experience of being
    mothered.

15 Ibid., p.156

16 Ibid., p.157

17 Ibid., p.158, Derrida's emphasis

18 Spivak, G.C. Translator's preface. In ibid., p.lxxvii

19 Thompson, D. A response to Gary Rolfe, *Nurse Education Today*,
    202, 22, pp.271-2; Watson, R. Faking an argument, *Nurse
    Education Today*, 2002, 22, pp.273-4

20 Rolfe, G. A response to Thompson and Watson, *Nurse Education
    Today*, 2002, 22, pp.275-7.

Faking a Difference: Evidence-Based
Nursing and the Illusion of Diversity

I will think about it
(this is the title)

'I'll teach you differences.'
King Lear
William Shakespeare

The politics of difference

'Diversity', in common with terms such
as 'community' and 'equality', is usually
taken to be a good thing almost without question. Diversity implies variety

There are many ways by
which one text can refer
to another, including:
'parody, pastiche, echo,
allusion, direct quota-
tion and structural
parallelism'[1]. This
Intertextuality, according to some theorists,
is the very condition of

(which, we are told, is the spice of life), deviation from dull routine, and eccentricity (in its safe 'English' form). For ecologists, biodiversity and an extended gene pool are signs of a healthy biosphere, whilst most sociologists argue that racial and cultural diversity are signs of a healthy society. And in everyday life, we all wish to assert our individuality, our divergence from the norm; no one wishes to be thought of as a conformist.

However, there is one sphere of activity where diversity is largely unwelcome, and that is in politics (in the broadest sense of the word). It is far easier to control or govern a convergent group; a group which thinks the same thoughts in the same way, believes in the same values, worships the same god(s), and even dresses in the same clothes (why else do certain groups such as soldiers and schoolchildren wear uniforms?). The political Right has always openly acknowledged this fear of diversity: the very word 'Conservative' suggests a certain restrained uniformity, and we need look no further than the penchant of the extreme Right for uniforms and its xenophobic, homophobic and even gynaephobic attitudes to confirm our suspicions. The political Left has a much finer tightrope to walk, since it has traditionally espoused an outward-looking, inclusive, devolutionary and internationalist attitude that mitigates against centralised rule. However, we can see in issues such as trade unionism and the rise of 'New Labour' how even the Left expects conformity and uniformity (and the ruthless ways in which it goes about enforcing it) when it

literature; all texts are woven from other texts whether their authors know it or not. But, whilst a text might assimilate or exploit earlier works of literature and point to areas of convergence, the author is invariably using such texts to add resonance or structure to their own *different* and *diverse* viewpoint on a given topic. Thus, whilst R is concerned with the 'seduction' of *assimilating* (using and evaporating) F's contribution into his own supplement (structure) with its inherent rules and language games, F is concerned with the Intertextuality of her own supplementary annotations and that of R's paper. That both the original deconstructive thesis (R's paper) and the supplement (F's deconstruction) are separate and yet woven together through Intertextuality is a fundamental starting point for a supplementary text which focuses on diversity, convergence, exclusion and inclusion. Perhaps then, this supplement is the 'real' fake, in that it is not different at all, but a parody; an exaggeration and an imitated illusion of difference.

comes to matters of power and control. The problem for the managers of broad-Left, liberal democratic organisations, then, is to be seen to be encouraging diversity of thought, belief and action, whilst maintaining the necessary conformity for trouble-free rule.

This is the dilemma faced not only by managers of seemingly liberal organizations such as schools, universities and (some) businesses, but also by larger and more nebulous entities such as academic disciplines and professional groups. All professions, by definition, are regulated. Entry to, and expulsion from, professional groups is controlled by a very small number of (sometimes) elected individuals who are charged with maintaining the credibility and standing of the profession both with its members and, more importantly, with the general public who (directly or indirectly) employ those professionals to provide a service. In maintaining internal and external credibility, it generally suits the professions to exude an air of liberal diversity, offering a range of roles and job opportunities to meet the requirements of all their potential members, and a range of services to meet the needs of all their potential clients. Even the traditionally convergent professions such as the armed forces and the police are seeking (perhaps half-heartedly) to diversify their membership to other cultural and ethnic groups such as homosexuals and black people in order to sustain or rebuild the confidence of their members and of the general public.

However, the task of regulating and controlling the professions calls for

Allusion

The early passing reference to the term community is, for me, an irresistible hook. The term, commonly associated with diversity, is fraught with preconceptions and is a potent word that obscures particularity, is overlaid with generalisations, idealisations, and abstractions. In this sense, it has more similarities with the concept of diversity than it has differences. According to Sardello the primary problem with the notion of community is the associated beliefs, namely that community can accomplish something that individuals alone cannot achieve. He says: 'We hear so much today about what people can do if they band together as a community – they can solve neighbourhood violence, get rid of unwanted elements, work together for their own improvement, take matters into their own hands when the system ignores the real needs of the people and become recognised as a force that cannot be ignored'[2]. This 'banding together' necessitates some sort of convergence of opinions, beliefs, values within the community, and again this is

different criteria from those required to maintain credibility. Divergence results in difference, and whereas a tolerance of difference is a useful attribute for promoting the public face of the profession, a degree of convergence towards uniformity is necessary for ensuring internal discipline and conformity. We have seen that, for professions such as the armed forces and the police, such convergence is overt and expected, and is enforced and demonstrated by the wearing of uniforms, parade drill, and unquestioning obedience. In other professions, such as education and law, the exercise of pressure to converge is far more subtle and often goes unrecognised by many of the members until they wittingly or unwittingly step over the often invisible boundaries.

Nursing, of course, started out as an overtly convergent profession, and still retains many of the trappings such as uniforms (usually with stripes, 'pips' or colour-coding to denote seniority) and overt hierarchies of command. However, it wishes more and more to be seen as a liberal profession (see, for example, the recent government paper, perhaps significantly entitled *Making a Difference*[1]) in which its members are seen to be thinking, autonomous and questioning practitioners and in which promotion depends on original thought and innovative practice rather than conformity to certain arcane standards of moral and social behaviour. My aim in this paper is to demonstrate that behind the liberal facade of diversity and the promotion of difference lies a core value of convergent conformism that serves to

thought to be a healthy sign. Yet, individuals within the community also strive for difference, for individuality. Herein lies a dilemma, for whilst diversity and community (which involves a degree of conformity) are deemed to be indicators of a healthy individual functioning in a healthy society, organisation or group, both are also seemingly in opposition.

Do individuals really want to be different? If we all conform to being diverse then we are not different at all, although conforming to difference may create a more conducive environment for a 'functional' community. Diversity, then, may be assimilated in the move towards community, in the basic desire to band together, experience inclusion and to be part of something bigger. Perhaps F would have preferred the experience of commune-ity implied in the '*subsuming*' of her contribution to R's paper, as opposed to the experience of diversifying and acknowledging her difference. Acknowledging one's difference, as an individual, means becoming visible and being seen as separate from others; peering above the para-

constrain individuality and stifle creativity.

Nursing, like most disciplines/professions, is characterised by a number of competing discourses, where a discourse is taken to be a set of rules or assumptions for organizing and interpreting the subject matter of an academic discipline or field of study[2]. Discourses are similar to what Kuhn[3] referred to as paradigms, and regulate matters such as which research methodologies are considered the most appropriate for generating knowledge in the discipline, how that knowledge is disseminated and taught, which kinds of projects receive funding, how practice should be organised, and on what kinds of knowledge it should be based. In nursing, the competing discourses include the medical model of practice, holism, reflective practice, evidence-based practice (EBP), and so on. There are clearly areas of overlap between these discourses, but each has its own methods, ideology, and criteria against which good practice is measured.

Generally speaking, one particular discourse dominates a discipline at any one time, and I suggest that a broadly medical model prevails in nursing, supported and funded by the Department of Health, and driven by innovations from the discipline of medicine such as EBP and the randomised controlled trial (RCT). In fact, as a general rule of thumb, the dominant discourse can usually be spotted simply by the fact that it does not need to justify itself. For example, you might have noticed that many qualitative research papers and dissertations begin with a discussion

pet and risking being known. More importantly, where professional practice is concerned, acknowledging ones difference is linked to intentional practice, in which the practitioner is not only responsible and accountable for their own practice, but also interested in where it meets and differs from that of others. But diversity requires its own convergence of opinions and beliefs, contains its own language games and rules and as such is no different to any other meta-narrative, albeit a meta-narrative that professes tolerance and inclusion and an acceptance of difference and particularity (and in this way alludes to the death of the meta-narrative).

What happens when others view the individuals who have 'banded together' as extremists (as can be seen in the current international situation 'waging war on terrorism')? Individuals banded together within a community may also continue to experience themselves as separate; people who are perceived as different to other members of society often come together, not necessarily because they agree with one another,

(and often a defence) of why a qualitative methodology was chosen, but that papers reporting on quantitative studies simply take as given that theirs is the method of choice.

Being a subscriber to the dominant discourse carries with it certain obvious privileges such as power, money and fame. Thus, if you practice, teach or research within the constraints of the dominant discourse, you are more likely to be promoted to a position of power and influence, you are more likely to be awarded grants for continuing and disseminating your work, and you are more likely to become a nationally recognised figure within your discipline. As might be expected, competition between discourses is fierce, and once power is attained it is generally clung to at all costs. Other discourses are demeaned and the power structure is re-organised in such a way that makes it difficult for the dominant discourse to be toppled. Kuhn describes how advocates of the dominant paradigm respond to challenges to it:

> Though they may begin to lose faith and then to consider alternatives, they do not renounce the paradigm that has led them into crisis. They do not, that is, treat anomalies as counter instances, though in the vocabulary of the philosophy of science that is what they are.... They will devise numerous articulations and *ad hoc* modifications of their theory in order to eliminate any apparent conflict.[4]

In nursing, for example, the dominant discourse has redefined research

but because what they have in common is that they are separate. Hence the 'outsiders' come together to form a group of 'insiders', but continue to remain 'outsiders'. How, I wonder, does this relate to nursing, and in particular to the different branches and specialisms within nursing, to qualitative researchers, and indeed to F and R?

We are presented here with an interesting dilemma regarding the degree of difference that can be tolerated within a community and indeed the inherent relationship between difference and deviance. When communities of individuals deviate from the dominant discourse about what is an acceptable and tolerable degree of diversity, a question emerges about the limits of the tolerance of diversity and how a community can achieve a 'common' stance in relation to these limits, that is, deciding what is and is not included. This notion of commonality fits better with the dictionary definition of community: 'All the people living in a specific locality; body of people having a religion, a profession etc in common'[3]. The word

us 'rigorous and systematic enquiry ... designed to lead to generalisable contributions to knowledge' in which 'small scale projects should be curbed'[5]. In this way, research which makes general statements about large populations based on quantitative statistical studies with large samples and experimental or quasi-experimental designs is favoured over qualitative research, much of which is small-scale and not widely generalisable, and therefore often falls outside the definition of what counts as research. Similarly, best practice has been rebadged as 'evidence-based' with the 'gold standard' of evidence being the RCT[6], so that practice not based on the findings of RCTs is, by definition, inferior.

But as we have seen, the dominant discourse has to be seen to be encouraging diversity, even though the consequences of diversity would inevitably lead to a dilution of the power, authority and dominance of that discourse. We therefore see a rhetoric of 'tolerance', of 'sharing', and most insidious of all, of 'assimilation', in which supporters of the dominant medical model discourse grudgingly acknowledge that competing discourses might have something useful to offer the discipline, whilst at the same time relegating the contribution from these competing discourses to a subservient role.

Deconstruction

In order to demonstrate how the dominant discourse appears to tolerate (and even encourage) diversity whilst at the same time acting to close it down, I shall offer a deconstructive reading of

'community' itself is derived from the Latin *communitas*, which is related to the word common. A community, then, as usually understood, defines itself by being against other aspects of the world and gains power by gathering together numbers of conforming individuals with a sense of commonality.

However, no matter how inclusive a group or community might be, it defines itself in relation to what does not belong, enforcing exclusion criteria through some sort of regulation.

Echoes

'If you must have values, celebrate difference and otherness. Structures and systems force us into sameness. Recognize the undecidability and openness of the world, its capacity always to become other'[4].

After many years of working within the counselling and psychotherapy field I decided it was time to apply for accreditation to the British Association for Counselling. I was working in General Practice as a clinical counsellor and motivated by the increasing pressure to join a professional body for counselling (become

three elements of EBP. Deconstruction is usually associated with the post-structuralist philosophers, particularly with the work of Jacques Derrida, and offers a powerful method of critiquing texts by exposing the contradictions and *aporia* that are inevitably written into them. Much of the activity of deconstruction therefore takes place in what Derrida[7] referred to as the 'margins of the text', in the seemingly innocuous and even superfluous passages where the author's guard is down. As Norris tells us:

> To "deconstruct" a piece of writing is therefore to operate a kind of strategic reversal, seizing on precisely those unregarded details (casual metaphors, footnotes, incidental turns of argument) which are always, and necessarily, passed over by interpreters of a more orthodox persuasion.[8]

It must be borne in mind, however, that there are as many deconstructive readings of a text as there are writers, and that each deconstruction is itself open to further deconstructions. This, then, is a single 'reading' of EBP that is no more or less privileged than any other reading.

Deconstructing the discourse of evidence-based practice

For Derrida[9], the notion of a text went far beyond a simple written manuscript to encompass all possible means of expression, including the spoken and the enacted. I shall begin, however, by focussing on several journal papers by writers who hold positions of power and

a member of a recognised club and join a community). The British Association for Counselling (now BACP), like the UKCC and the UKCP, are in the security business; they protect the public by appointing people to act as external regulators of professions that advocate autonomous self-regulating professionals. What these individuals (and therein the professional bodies) actually regulate is not practice; rather they audit the ability of the professional to self-regulate. In this sense the practitioners are assessed on their ability to respond to external surveillance. One might question if such assessments/audits are representative of the diversity of practitioners and their practice: what information is really captured in the regulation of professionals? I believe it is the ability of the practitioner to conform. Which of course, in general, they do, but they also find ways of subverting the professional regulators. Witness the number of professional portfolios that sit gathering dust on shelves. Professional regulation is one way of

influence in the dominant discourse, and who therefore have most to gain in perpetuating the discourse and most to lose by its demise. I intend to demonstrate the contradiction implicit in many of these texts in respect to the issue of diversity, in particular, how the public face of EBP attempts to promote the illusion of diversity whilst the hidden agenda is to close it down.

In fact, many of these contradictions are quite overt and explicit; they are on the surface of the text for all to see. For example, the paper by the self-styled 'Evidence-Based Medicine Working Group' (EBMWG), which originally launched evidence-based medicine, stated boldly that:

> Evidence-based medicine de-emphasises intuition, unsystematic clinical experience, and pathophysiologic rationale as sufficient grounds for clinical decision making.[10]

Thus, only in cases where there is a 'dearth of adequate evidence' or where certain 'aspects of clinical practice cannot, or will not, ever be adequately tested'[11] should we fall back on other forms of evidence such as intuition and clinical experience. On this reading, then, EBP is clearly *against* divergence: it de-emphasises the intuition and clinical experience of individual practitioners in favour of evidence based on the self-proclaimed 'gold standard' of RCTs. The very existence of a gold standard mitigates against diversity, and the last thing that is wanted is for individual practitioners to be making clinical decisions according to their own individual judgements.

standardising diversity, of attending to the need to demonstrate both diversity and conformity (both indicators of credibility) within public services.

I dutifully completed my forms, in duplicate of course, including a portfolio of evidence collected over a period of 10 years. As advised, I contacted other accredited counsellors, who for a fee offered their critical reading of my application. I paid a further fee to have my application assessed and I waited until the next formal meeting of the accreditation panel. My application was rejected; I received no feedback as to why. I was given no indication of what I needed to do in order to be accepted by the club, just that I was not fit to be a member. What were my options? To conform, that is, to find a way to subscribe to the dominant discourse; to subscribe to the dominant discourse and subvert it; to start a discourse of my own, risking marginalization (which in fact was no risk as I had already been marginalized by BAC). In fact I move between all three: I have found a way to subscribe to the dominant

Indeed, many later writers made this convergent attitude towards practice absolutely explicit. Thus, French interpreted EBP as 'The process of systematic identification, rigorous evaluation and the subsequent dissemination of the use of the findings of research to influence clinical practice'[12], and continued by adding that 'the gold standard for evaluating the effectiveness of an intervention is the randomised controlled trial'[13]. This sentiment is echoed by DiCenso et al, who asserted that 'evidence-based health care is about applying the best available evidence to a specific clinical question'[14], and qualified that statement by adding that 'the RCT is the most appropriate design for evaluating the effectiveness of a nursing intervention'[15]. The message could not be clearer: as far as possible, all nursing interventions should be based *not* on the expert clinical judgement of the experienced nurse, but on the findings of RCTs.

One reading of the imposition of a 'gold standard' is that it ensures the quality of the nursing intervention. An alternative reading, however, is that it serves to exert control over practitioners by ensuring that they all respond in the same way to the same clinical situation. In effect, it minimizes choice on the premise that all practitioners are essentially interchangeable (in other words, that they are identical). Although such a strategy might serve to regulate practice, the suppression (or de-emphasis) of individual clinical judgement in favour of research evidence is likely to alienate large numbers of practitioners, particularly those who regard themselves as experts. Thus, in the very same

discourse and conform to professional regulation by becoming an accredited member of the UKCP; however, I continue to subvert the role and discourses of professional bodies through such activities as deconstruction and discourse analysis, which in effect, helps me to construct a discourse of my own. Thus, I find a way to conform and belong, whilst simultaneously maintaining my difference, although not always openly.

As you may expect then, the inherent politics of disguised liberalism and the continued marginalization of practice knowledge resonates deeply with my own experience of the rhetoric of diversity and subsequent tokenism. The type of disguised liberalism that R refers to in his thesis is very seductive, not least because those espousing it are often very charismatic in their approach and persuasive in their arguments. With oppression masquerading as liberalism it is hard to know who the enemy is (if indeed there is one) and what their motivation might be, aside from the power and authority that accompany

paper that de-emphasised intuition and clinical experience as suitable forms of evidence, we are informed that 'clinical experience and the development of clinical instincts ... are a crucial and necessary part of becoming a competent physician'[16].

Similarly, later papers also acknowledge 'clinical expertise' as a valid form of evidence[17,18,19], although we can detect some reluctance and ambivalence in this acknowledgement. Thus, DiCenso et al appear keen to include the clinical judgement of the nurse in the equation, stating that 'clinical expertise must prevail if the nurse decides that the patient is too frail for a specific intervention that is otherwise "best" for his condition'[20]. However, they elsewhere flatly contradict this stance, stating that:

> We strongly disagree with White's assertion [that expertise is a better basis for clinical decision making than the RCT]. History has shown numerous examples of healthcare interventions which, on a patient by patient basis, might appear to be beneficial, but when evaluated using randomised trials have been shown to be of doubtful value, or even harmful.[21]

It is possible that the writers were unaware of their contradictory statements: that intuition and clinical experience should be both 'de-emphasised' and 'play a crucial role in becoming a competent physician'[22]; and that clinical expertise 'must prevail' whilst at the same time being 'of doubtful value, or even harmful'[23]. On this reading, they

fame and influence.

Parody

'*Paradoxically, she celebrates difference, not by differentiating, but by accepting every aspect of the environment as being of equal value*'[5].

One might usefully question what the motivating factors are for someone like R to write this paper. It is a paper that seemingly deconstructs and subverts, or attempts to subvert, the dominant discourse of evidence-based medicine and in particular its disguised liberalism in assimilating practitioner-based experience into its hierarchy of evidence model. More importantly, R's paper warns of the perils of being seduced into a community with which the practitioner has less in common than they have difference and where the price to pay for inclusion is a loss of imagination, autonomy, independence and creativity[6]. As R points out, difference is superficially accepted and assimilated into the discourse of evidence-based medicine, tolerated for the sake of placating, potentially, a multitude of powerful

were simply asserting the natural tendency of *any* dominant discourse towards practice based on a single and easily controlled precept (in this case, the RCT), whilst at the same time exuding a veneer of tolerance, divergence, and acceptance of individual clinical decisions.

A second reading, however, is that the contradictory statements represent a cynical exercise in what the postmodern architect Charles Jencks has called 'double coding', in which two different messages for two different audiences are simultaneously promulgated in the same text. Double coding entails a 'radical schizophrenia' that 'confirms and subverts simultaneously'[24]. In this case, the message to practitioners is that EBP continues to value their traditional skills and experience, whereas the message to academics is that the skills of conducting and critiquing research are the most valuable. In this way, academics are able to exert power over practitioners by concealing the 'true' nature of EBP. As Foucault pointed out, 'Power is tolerable only on condition that it mask a substantial part of itself. Its success is proportional to its ability to hide its own mechanisms'[25].

David Thompson, then Professor of Nursing Research at the Department of Health (and therefore firmly entrenched in the dominant discourse), moves beyond contradiction and concealment to outright denial in his paper entitled 'Why evidence-based nursing'[26]. From the deconstructionist's point of view, it is worth dwelling briefly on the title, which is another subtle example of double coding. On first

and alternative discourses.

But how do we know that R is not also faking his intolerance and difference to the dominant discourse of EBM? In classical rhetorical style, and to use the postmodern term 'aporia' in the troubling of R's text, how do we know his doubt regarding EBM, and of diversity, is real or pretend. Is R pretending to be diverse because diversity, as he points out, is thought to be a good thing? Further, is he conforming to the rules of a game, which, it would appear, he advocates opting out of? Or perhaps the aim of R's text is not to be diverse, but to be autonomous? R, it would seem, like all of us, struggles with conformity and diversity. R writes of the difficulty of being published within certain journals, unless of course one is firmly embedded within the positivist tradition; can R, or indeed any of us wishing to be published, afford to be too extreme in his views? The desire to be included in the academic community through activities such as writing dictates, to some extent, the level of difference (and separate-

glance, the title is democratic, inclusive and exudes an air of toleration of difference, suggesting a debate around the question of why we might adopt the practice of evidence-based nursing. Note, however, the absence of a question mark; the title is not posing a question, but outlining an imperative. Thompson is not *asking* 'why should we adopt evidence-based nursing?', but *asserting* 'this is why we should adopt it'. Under the veneer of divergence lies the rhetoric of convergence.

This suspicion is confirmed by the content of the paper, which begins with the usual reassurances that 'evidence-based healthcare, including nursing, is about integrating research evidence with clinical expertise, the resources available and the views of patients'[27]. However, the entire paper is then devoted to discussing strategies for implementing *research*, and interestingly, the words 'clinical expertise' are never again mentioned. The public face of EBP is inclusive; we can all contribute to the evidence required for best practice. However, the underlying message is that the only 'real' evidence comes from research, and even then, as we shall later show, not from the sort of research that practitioners might become involved in.

We can begin to see, then, that the way that EBP addresses the problem of diversity is by assimilation of competing discourses. Alternative forms of evidence such as expertise and clinical experience are seemingly welcomed, but at the same time are demeaned and discounted as 'blind conjecture, dogmatic ritual or private intuition'[28].

ness) that R can make visible.

If the aim of the R's text, as we are led to believe, is that of deconstructing EBM's disguised tolerance of difference, then I believe he achieves this. Deconstruction involves turning things upside down, making the hitherto oppressed side the dominating one. However, to deconstruct R's deconstruction, whilst he prises open the text of EBM, this is only the first step. The next step of deconstruction moves beyond the inversion of a hierarchy between two opposite sides, undermining 'the difference between the two opposites' as well as displacing 'the whole opposition in favour of another notion'[7]. Hence 'the first step involves a deconstruction of the previously dominating picture, in favour of what was hidden, dominated. The second step involves a deconstruction of both these poles, but at the same time a displacement of them, and thus a construction of something new and wider, in which the two at most constitute a special case[8]. Could R's last statement 'we must all, then, become philosophers' be construed as

Deconstructing the hierarchy of research evidence

There is a general consensus within the dominant discourse of EBP that the RCT is the 'gold standard' of research evidence, but that other methodologies, including qualitative approaches, have a role to play. Thus, DiCenso et al claim that:

> We hope to convey that good evidence does involve more than RCTs and systematic overviews. Each research design has its purpose, its strengths, and its limitations. The key is ensuring that the right research design is used to answer the question posed.[29]

Thus, whereas the RCT is the gold standard for evaluating clinical interventions, 'qualitative studies are the best designs to better understand patients' experiences, attitudes, and beliefs'[30]. The public face of evidence-based practice is therefore of an inclusive strategy that simply matches the best design to the question being asked. We might expect, then, that problems such as 'understanding patients suffering and how that suffering can be ameliorated by the caring and compassionate physician'[31] would be just the sort of question to be addressed by a qualitative methodology. However, the writers continue by stating that:

> The new paradigm [of EBP] would call for using the techniques of behavioural science to determine what patients are really looking for from their physicians and how

the beginning of something new and wider?

R asked F to contribute to the paper, perhaps demonstrating his commitment to diversity and to his philosophy. And when this is no longer possible, he invites F to write a supplement. Hence, rather than impose a single vision or monologic interpretation on the world of evidence-based medicine/nursing, he opts for a dialogic viewpoint, which as it were, talks to each other (in this case R and F), and indeed to other voices outside the text (you the reader). R points out that EBM is a monologic interpretation of the world of practice, and whilst its advocates espouse the benefits of dialogue, the discourse is, in fact, not open for discussion[9]. However, even the dialogic viewpoint is a partial view, making no recourse to holism.

Allusion

People, and that includes nurses, medics and the current authors, are locked into their research paradigms, locked into their particular and partial views about the nature of knowledge as evidenced by

physician and patient behaviour affects the outcome of care. Ultimately, randomised controlled trials using different strategies for interacting with patients ... may be appropriate.[32]

It appears that even issues such as patients' attitudes towards their care are best answered through the RCT, and only 'when definitive evidence [from RCTs] is not available one must fall back on weaker evidence'[33]. This suspicion is supported in the writing of Kevin Gournay, a nurse researcher and influential figure with the Department of Health, who, with Sue Ritter, argues that:

There is of course a place for qualitative methods, but such research needs to use a rigorous approach *and should be linked to quantitative methodologies ... for it to have any meaning.*[34]

I am suggesting, then, that beneath the rhetoric of diversity of methodology, of the most suitable method for each research question, lies a barely disguised contempt for methodologies from competing discourses as 'weaker forms of evidence' which only have meaning when linked to quantitative studies. Furthermore, such a strategy of ordering research in a hierarchy has two distinct benefits for the dominant discourse.

First, in becoming assimilated into the discourse of EBP, qualitative research paradigms are tacitly agreeing to abide by the criteria of quantitative research, criteria such as generalisability, validity and rigour that

their choice of research methodology. Yet, nurses generally do not think about the nature of knowledge, swept up as they are in a modernist view, dominated by methodological imperialism.

Even after 30 years of post-modernism's relentless critique of the modernist view, nurse researchers still cling to an essentially modernist view, perhaps because we lack the conviction to emerge from the shadows, as already mentioned, to be seen to be different (to be known as the expert). Paradoxically nurses are gasping for research that is meaningful for themselves as practitioners and for their everyday practice. The modernist view, to know a thing in itself in order to control and predict the world, is even evident in the shift to the so-called 'qualitative' paradigm. Embracing qualitative methods, however, does not shift the essential modernist mind-set, which is masked by moving from statistical correlation to using words; the effort is still to know the thing in itself.

Perhaps the shift from quantitative-type methodologies to qualitative-type methodologies

condemn them forever as second-class methodologies. Gournay and Ritter are quite clear on the criteria by which qualitative studies should be judged:

> We do not accept that scientific rigour is achieved by an interviewer who has not undergone interobserver reliability testing, or by validity testing that does not include a description of the constructs under consideration and that does not include test-retest data, or by use of terms such as 'symbolic interactionalism' in an article that makes no reference to Mead.[35]

Interobserver reliability and test-retest reliability are both criteria of quantitative research instruments, and have little or no meaning for qualitative researchers. Indeed, it is difficult even to imagine how we might go about measuring the interobserver reliability of an in-depth interview or the test-retest reliability of a set of observational field notes.

Such a naive understanding of issues of validity and reliability in qualitative research might be laughed off were it not for the fact of Gournay's pre-eminent influence with both the nursing hierarchy and the Department of Health. Apart from demonstrating a shocking ignorance of even the basics of qualitative research design, we would accept his argument that all articles on symbolic interactionism should mention G.H. Mead if and when all articles on RCTs (including Gournay's own work) mention Ronald Fisher as the founder of RCT methodology. But as we argued earlier, the dominant discourse

reflected an uneasy sense in nurses that modernism was alienating, that there was something intrinsically uncaring about such research that attempted to manipulate people as objects. Research on caring needs itself to be caring. Such congruence would seem to be fundamental. Yet, words have simply replaced numbers and perhaps people experience less contradiction and incongruence. Hence, the phenomenologist still takes an 'objective' stance, she brackets, otherwise her research is tarnished by the stain of bias. The illusion that self (which in itself is an illusion) can be objective is astonishing. Perhaps even more astonishing is the claim that phenomenology can adequately represent lived experience. It portrays, and in portraying life as fragmentary yet unproblematic, snippets of text are used as 'evidence' to support a largely arbitrary set of themes that somehow portray meaning. Yet such work does offer partial views that are useful to inform the practitioner – but only that – the risk, in our lingering modern world is that practitioners

has no need to justify its basic assumptions and first principles.

Second, by ordering research into a hierarchy in which the gold standard is the large-scale (and therefore expensive) RCT rather than the small-scale qualitative study (which might not require any external funding), the dominant discourse is able to maintain a tight control over what is researched and who is to research it. Not only does the government and its various agencies control the purse strings to most of the major research grants, thereby determining who will be funded to carry out the large-scale 'gold standard' research studies, but certain influential nurse researchers are also attempting to define what counts as adequate research training and who is competent to carry it out. Thus, Kevin Gournay and Sue Ritter, writing specifically about psychiatric nurse researchers, claimed that 'A priority is to establish an infrastructure of properly trained researchers'[36]. For Gournay and Ritter, 'properly trained' means having a doctoral qualification, although:

> When one scrutinizes PhD theses written by psychiatric nurses, many are based on qualitative and uncontrolled studies. To compound the problem there appears to be a considerable variation in pass standards for PhDs between universities, and some theses contain fundamental flaws of design, analysis and write up.[37]

Not just any PhD will do. It should be conducted in an approved (by Gournay and Ritter) university using an and people are fitted into such systems in our efforts to know and control the world.

Was grasping hermeneutics the answer to this further disquiet? Now we can stop pretending to be objective and say we must pay attention to ourselves as researchers in what we do - it is okay, in fact fashionable, to be subjective - to see the other through a lens of our own bias, as long as this is made explicit. More honesty, less contradiction - yet not fundamentally changing the style of research.

Nevertheless, standing in judgement of the modernist mind-set in relation to research is to fall into the same trap of offering yet another partial view, getting caught up in the dogma and intolerance to other views that such partiality nurtures. What happens to the indefinite deferral of judgement? And yet, such judgment is fundamental to the current activity of deconstruction. As such, each one of us needs to see that we are locked into partial views, including R and F. The task is to notice where we have invested our energy, what our reputations and identities cling to, and the

approved (by Gournay and Ritter) methodology.

The philosopher Jean-François Lyotard referred to this strategy of judging all discourses according to the rules and criteria of the most powerful as a *differend*, which is 'a case of conflict between (at least two) parties that cannot be equitably resolved for lack of a rule applicable to both arguments'[38]. It is clearly a situation in which power takes precedence over knowledge, and 'a wrong results from the fact that the rules of the genre of discourse by which one judges are not those of the judged genre or genres of discourse'[39]. We can see in the above example, then, that once qualitative researchers allow themselves to become sucked into the hierarchy of evidence, they will inevitably find themselves on the wrong end of a *differend*, and will quickly become marginalised.

Deconstructing the journal 'Evidence-Based Nursing'

We turn now from written texts to a deconstruction of a journal. 'Evidence-Based Nursing' is edited by Alba DiCenso, Nicky Cullum and Donna Ciliska, whose paper I cited above. All are key players in the evidence-based nursing movement: DiCenso and Ciliska are at McMaster University in Canada, from where evidence-based medicine originated, and Cullum is at the Centre for Evidence-Based Nursing at the University of York, which has close links with the Department of Health (DoH), and where David Thompson, Professor of Nursing Research at the DoH, was also based. The journal, then, can be

extent to which we are more concerned with self-interest (even in the belonging to the 'right' club) than any form of dialogue or concern with practice. As Fox comments: 'Research should be *constitutive* of *difference*, rather than *constitutive* of *identity*[10].

Maybe, as R points out, it is all a matter of language. That is to say that language is everything and nothing. That the term 'evidence' for example, a single word, should serve as the inflated focus for such a range of contradictory investments renders it both potent and serves to make it an invalid or meaningless concept. But what is missed in the debating of the meaning of a word is that the degree of semantic complexity surrounding the term might signal the fact that 'a significant number of people with conflicting interests and opinions feel that there is something sufficiently important at stake here worth struggling and arguing over'[11].

So, rather than offer two different messages for two different audiences, this chapter offers two different and similar messages for the

seen as an international mouthpiece of the dominant discourse. As such, my contention is that part of the remit of the journal is to maintain control and influence over practice, and to curb the proliferation of competing discourses in favour of a convergence towards practice based on the self-professed 'gold standard' of RCTs.

My suggestion that the journal achieves this convergence towards a narrow and easily controlled mode of practice by controlling the flow of evidence on which practice is to be based, is perhaps borne out by examining the aims of the journal, which are published on page 2 of every issue. Here we see that the journal aims 'to identify ... the best ... articles', 'to summarise this literature in the form of structured abstracts', 'to provide brief, highly expert comment...' and 'to disseminate the summaries in a timely fashion to nurses'. Nurses no longer need to choose which papers to read, to assess them for themselves, and to engage in debate over their strengths and weaknesses. Indeed, they do not need to read original papers at all, merely to digest summaries of papers selected for them as being 'best'. Neither do they need to critically assess them, since each summary is accompanied by 'brief, highly expert comment'.

There are a number of points to be made about these objectives. Firstly, most academic journals aim to promote debate and discussion. For example, *Nurse Education Today* 'acts as an interface between the theory and practice of nurse education, stimulating change and cross-fertiliza-

same audience, providing two partial views, which we feel are worth struggling over.

Pastiche and Direct Quotation

'The title of a novel is part of the text – the first part of it, in fact, we encounter - and therefore has considerable power to attract and condition the reader's attention'[12].

Referring to a paper written by Professor David Thompson, R writes:

> From the deconstructionist's point of view, it is worth dwelling briefly on the title, which is another subtle example of double coding. On first glance, the title is democratic, inclusive and exudes an air of toleration and difference, suggesting a debate around the question of why we might adopt the practice of evidence based nursing. Note, however, the absence of a question mark; the title is not posing a question, but outlining an imperative. Thompson is not *asking* 'why should we adopt evidence based nursing?' but *assert-*

tion of ideas', and the *Journal of Psychiatric and Mental Health Nursing* 'provides a forum for critical debate...'. Even *Clinical Effectiveness in Nursing*, which covers similar ground to *Evidence-Based Nursing*, seeks to interact both with its writers and its readers by offering 'peer commentary, to which the authors then respond in the same issue. A correspondence section is used to widen the debate'. *Evidence-Based Nursing*, however, has no such liberal aims. It does not seek to generate debate, but to disseminate highly selective information. It does not seek to stimulate its readers into questioning the findings it presents, but to provide a definitive assessment in the form of 'brief, highly expert comment'. In short, it neither elicits nor publishes a diversity of opinion, but rather conveys the message that such diversity is unnecessary and, indeed, even harmful.

It is interesting to note the extent to which the journal editors draw on authority and expertise in order to justify their aims. We have already seen that the abstracts published in the journal are validated by 'clinical experts'. Given that evidence-based medicine 'puts a much lower value on authority'[40], we might question the status of their 'highly expert comments'. Or perhaps it is only *clinical* expertise that has lost its authority and not the methodological expertise that is required to evaluate the research studies. Certainly, the editors appear to regard themselves as experts. In their paper 'Implementing evidence-based nursing: some misconceptions'[41], they claim to correct the 'misunderstandings'

ing 'this is why we should adopt it'. Under the veneer of divergence lies the rhetoric of convergence.

For the writer, choosing a title is an important part of the writing process, for as Lodge asserts, an 'indifference to naming' is a symptom of a loss of faith in one's vocation[13]. The title brings into sharper focus what the paper is supposed to be about. And so what of the title of R's paper?

The 'Faking a Difference' appears to be an (in)direct reference, perhaps even a parody, of the government document *Making a Difference*[14], which R refers to early on in his thesis. The term 'faking' belies a degree of cynicism and scepticism that becomes apparent as the reader enters the body of the thesis. Or perhaps R is referring to himself, telling the reader that his thesis is faking difference. Then there is the matter of the colon, a significant inclusion if we are to follow R's deconstruction of the exclusion of the question mark in Thompson's paper. What of the colon? According to the Oxford English Dictionary the colon is

surrounding evidence-based nursing in an authoritative way that seems calculated to narrow down the concept of evidence-based nursing rather than opening it up. By replacing the authority of the clinical expert with that of the methodological expert, decisions about what constitutes good practice are confined to a small group that is largely sympathetic to the dominant discourse of evidence (research) based practice. One reading of the aims of the journal *Evidence-Based Nursing* is therefore to shut down diversity of opinion by transferring the authority to make clinical decisions from the individual judgements of a large number of clinical experts to the consensual judgement of a much smaller number of hand-picked methodological experts, based on the 'predefined criteria' established by the journal itself.

Difference/*Différance*

I have argued that a healthy discipline requires a strategy for diversity that results not in an assimilation/absorption of the competition by the dominant discourse but in difference, that is, in a community of discourses that each play by their own rules, but on a level playing field where resources are allocated to projects which meet the criteria of their *own* discourse rather than those of the dominant discourse. Unfortunately, the entire edifice of rational Western thought mitigates against this ideal. The philosophy of realism/empiricism on which it is based argues that there is a single truth that corresponds to an external and unchanging reality. Furthermore, the

used: between two main clauses of which, the second explains, enlarges on, or follows from the first; to introduce a list of items; and before a quotation. R, I would argue, has used the colon to link (and indeed separate) the two main clauses of the paper, but what are they? The title is seductive in that it has several connotations, some more overt than others, which, depending on the reader, may or may not be of consequence.

Difference?

This paper ends with the bold statement that 'we must all become philosophers'. Indeed, we must, but philosophers of a certain kind, if we are to follow R's thesis: that is, *applied* philosophers. On the surface this appears to be yet another partial view and perhaps one might argue that in this sense R is no different from those subjects who are the focus of his arguments (Kevin Gournay and David Thompson for example). There are, however, I believe, several differences in the way that R presents his case, one of which relates to his willingness to deviate from and challenge the dominant discourses

method of science is usually recognised as the only way accurately to
gain access to that reality through
ruthlessly discarding theories when new
and 'better' ones come along. Thus,
Popper has argued that scientific
theories compete with one another in a
Darwinian sense, and that 'our knowledge consists, at every moment, of
those hypotheses which have shown
their (comparative) fitness by surviving
so far in their struggle for existence; a
competitive struggle which eliminates
those hypotheses which are unfit'[42]. In
nature, of course, such a strategy of
natural selection ensures not only the
elimination of species that cannot
adapt, but also the diversity and
proliferation of those that can. In
science, however, where the rules are
fixed to favour knowledge and theories
emanating from the dominant paradigm, what ensues is not diversity, but a
consolidation of the status quo and a
culture of 'conform or perish'.

True diversity cannot flourish in a
culture of competitiveness where the
rules are fixed by the most powerful
player, and in order to generate and
sustain difference, we require a strategy
not of assimilation/absorption, but of
différance[43]. The attitude of *différance*
was formulated by Derrida in the face
of the problem of how to accept conflicting discourses without becoming
drawn into the dispute between them.
The word *différance* is a combination
of the French words for difference and
deferral. It is therefore a neologism (or,
as Derrida prefers, a 'neographism',
since it can be distinguished from the
French word 'différence' only in its
written form), which takes on a mean-

around health services
research.

The notion of applied
philosophy is not new,
indeed a number of
contemporary researchers
regard the research
endeavour as one of
applied philosophy.
Bentz and Shapiro, for
example, believe that
the working researcher
is always a kind of
applied philosopher and
remind us that before
the 19th century the
sciences did not exist
as separate disciplines
but were a part of philo-
sophy. They go on to say
that:

> ...The author will say
> that research is about
> creating *science* or
> *knowledge* about the
> *world* or *reality* or
> *society* or *human
> behaviour*. But what is
> science? What is know-
> ledge? What is real-
> ity? These are
> precisely philosophic-
> al questions and any
> statement about them
> is a philosophical
> one[15].

Few would argue that
these fundamental
(philosophical) quest-
ions with their divers-
ity of responses are
central to the develop-
ment of any research
project. But surely what
is of utmost importance
(and to some extent an

ing of both (or, as Derrida would have it, of neither). As Sim points out, 'it is an alternative term for both unity *and* difference'[44]. To approach a dispute with an attitude of *différance*, then, is to accept the differences between the two sides but to defer indefinitely any attempt to choose between them, to transcend the very concept of polar opposites.

Derrida's strategy for dealing with *différance* was to put any word (signifier) whose concept (signified) invokes competing and unresolvable differences 'under erasure' *(sous rature)* by writing a cross over it. Thus, we might place the word 'evidence' under erasure by writing it as evidence. As Spivak observed, this denotes

> the mark of the absence of a presence, an always already absent present, of the lack at the origin that is the condition of thought and experience.[45]

By placing the signifier 'evidence' under erasure, we are signalling that it has no fixed signified, no origin. As a signifier of something in the world, it both exists and does not exist, and 'must make its necessity felt before letting itself be erased'[46]. The signifier evidence is now freed from any or all of its signifieds and its meaning can drift *(derive)* across and between discourses. Evidence can, at the same time and without contradiction, refer to the findings of an RCT, to the preferences expressed by patients, to the introspective thoughts of the reflective practitioner and to the intuition of the expert. But of course, it also refers to

indicator of success) to any researcher (at least in health sciences) is the extent to which it informs practice. R's position on this is one that we are left in little doubt about. Or perhaps he is faking it.

What is often most influential in the development of evidence-based nursing, as R alludes to, are the politics, the power dynamics and the degree of conformity (or inclusion). Politics are very influential in the construction of the social self and the construction of what constitutes deviance, difference and diversity. As already alluded to, the politics of deviance is a whole interesting area in itself and merits a deconstruction of its own. Whilst this is not the purpose of this paper, suffice it to say that any dominant discourse constructs the norm, and by default, defines the deviant. I, myself, am probably classed as one of the deviants, but as Groucho Marx once remarked, he didn't care to belong to a club that would accept people like himself as a member! Nevertheless, a sense of belonging is important and the balance between needing to be different and needing

none of these; it is a signifier without a signified, which as Lyotard observed, 'is in fact contradictory and not acceptable within the logic of identity'[48]. By writing it under erasure, the signifier evidence transcends the different meanings (signifieds) given to it by different discourses. Thus, whenever we come across the word, we must defer its meaning, we must think of it as having several contradictory meanings and no meaning at all. *Différance* therefore promotes diversity in a way that the rules of the dominant paradigm would never allow, indeed, in a way that the Aristotelian logic of 'either-or' explicitly forbids.

As we might imagine, the 'slipperiness' introduced by *différance* is generally unwelcome in academic discourses, since it suggests a certain laxity, imprecision and disregard for logic which most scientific disciplines would wish to move away from. However, we have already seen that for Lyotard, such a move away from the toleration of difference is motivated less by the desire for academic and scientific credibility than by the desire for power. Difference leads to dispute (a *differend*), and a *differend* implies a victory of power over knowledge. When academics defend certainty over uncertainty and 'gold standards' over local standards, they are merely defending their power base. As Lyotard observed, an intellectual is 'someone who helps forget *differends* ... for the sake of political hegemony'[49], as opposed to the philosopher who 'bear[s] witness to the *differend*' by exposing the inequality inherent in it.

to belong is a difficult one to negotiate. It is notoriously difficult for the agent to mediate their internal and external world, and even more difficult to deal with subtle conformity disguised as freedom and labelled diversity. The rhetoric about diversity, which R's paper clearly challenges us to deconstruct, is undermined by the sense of constant surveillance[16], which pervades nursing, nurse education and evidence-based practice. This deconstruction is of significance given that they all espouse autonomy and monitor this, yes - through surveillance!!

Echoes
Reading R's paper reminded me of the secret handshake societies and stimulated questions regarding which club practitioners align themselves with. Do they have any choice about membership? Perhaps, as R suggests, they can only get into certain clubs if they conform to the covert entrance criteria. Practitioners then should ask not only which club they would want to belong to, but also question whether they would want to belong to any club. But then if they opt out of

We must all, then, become philosophers.

Notes

1 Department of Health *Making a Difference*, London: DoH, 1999
2 Jenkins, K. *Re-Thinking History*, London: Routledge, 1991
3 Kuhn, T.S. *The Structure of Scientific Revolutions (3e)*, Chicago: The University of Chicago Press, 1996
4 Ibid., pp.77-8
5 Department of Health *Report of the Taskforce on the Strategy for Research in Nursing, Midwifery and Health Visiting*, London: DoH, 1993. P.13
6 Long, A.F. Health services research - a radical approach to cross the research and development divide. In M. Baker & S. Kirk (eds) *Research and Development for the NHS*, Oxon: Radcliffe Medical Press, 1998
7 Derrida, J. *Of Grammatology*, Baltimore: The Johns Hopkins University Press, 1976
8 Norris, C. *Derrida*, London: Fontana Press, 1987, p.19
9 Derrida, op.cit.
10 Evidence-Based Medicine Working Group. Evidence-based medicine: a new approach to teaching the practice of medicine, *JAMA*, 1992, 268, 17, 2420-5, p.2420
11 Ibid.
12 French, B. Developing the skills required for evidence-based practice, *Nurse Education Today*, 1998, 18, 46-51.
13 Ibid.
14 DiCenso A., Cullum N. & Ciliska D. Implementing evidence-based

being a member, they become, by default, members of another club and run the risk of being marginalised.

The question comes then: how we do encourage diversity, which encourages a sceptical stance in relation to diversity? This is where R's deconstruction comes in, but even deconstruction is a diversification requiring a cultural change and a tolerance of deferral of judgment. Is it really okay for practitioners to be different in a world of standardization and a culture of blame? The contradictions are rife: how can we enable practitioners to view evidence-based practice from a position of diversity when we have an essentialist education, where competencies for practice are standardized and there is a lack of diversity of evidence permitted in assignments (see, for example, portfolios which are usually assessed using a standard format and don't allow for such things as poetry, art and photo essays as evidence of best practice)? If nurses experience evidence-based practice as oppressive (and I only have personal experience

nursing: some misconceptions, *Evidence-Based Nursing*, 1998, 1, 2, 38-40.

15 Ibid.

16 EBMWG, op.cit.

17 Sackett, D.L., Rosenberg, W.M.C., Gray, J.A.M., Haynes, R.B. & Richardson, W.S. Evidence based medicine: what it is and what it isn't, *British Journal of Medicine*, 1996, 312, 71-2

18 DiCenso et al, op. cit.

19 Thompson, D. Why evidence based nursing, *Nursing Standard*, 1998, 13, 9, 58-9

20 DiCenso et al, op. cit.

21 Ibid., p.39

22 EBMWG, op.cit.

23 DiCenso et al, op. cit.

24 Jencks, C. *What is Post-Modernism?* (4e), Chichester: John Wiley, 1996, p.30

25 Foucault, M. *The History of Sexuality: An Introduction*, Harmondsworth: Penguin, 1976, p.71

26 Thompson, D. op. cit.

27 Ibid.

28 Blomfield, R & Hardy, S. Evidence-based nursing practice. In L. Trinder & S. Reynolds (eds) *Evidence-Based Practice: A Critical Approach*, Oxford: Blackwell Science, 2000, p.4

29 DiCenso, op. cit., p.39

30 Ibid.

31 EBMWG, op. cit.

32 Ibid., p.2422

33 Ibid.

34 Gournay, K. & Ritter, S. What future for research in mental health nursing?, *Journal of Psychiatric and Mental Health Nursing*, 1997, 4, 441-6, p.442, my emphasis

35 Gournay, K. & Ritter, S. What future

to suggest that this might be the case), little wonder that some adopt a separatist approach, undermining the implementation of such directives as 'clinical guidelines'. Isn't this what people like Gournay want? If the masses are split then they are less powerful and easier to control and manipulate; a critical mass is more difficult to achieve if there is no cohesive voice, even one that espouses diversity.

Notes

1   Lodge, D. *The Art of Fiction*, London: Penguin, 1992, p.98

2   Sardello, R. *Love and the Soul. Creating a future for Earth*, New York: Harper Collins, 1995, p.187

3   *Oxford Compact English Dictionary*, Oxford: Oxford University Press, 1996

4   Fox, N.J. *Beyond Health: Postmodernism and Embodiment*, London: Free Association Books, 1999, p.96

5   Ibid., p.178

6   Okri, B. *A way of being Free*, London: Phoenix, 1997

7   Alvesson, M. and Skoldberg, K. *Reflexive Methodol-*

for research in mental health nursing: a rejoinder to Parsons, Beech and Rolfe, *Journal of Psychiatric and Mental Health Nursing*, 1998, 5, 227-230, p.228

36 Gournay & Ritter, 1997, op. cit.

37 Ibid., p.441

38 Lyotard, J-F. *The Differend: Phrases in Dispute*, Minneapolis: University of Minnesota Press, 1983, p.xi

39 Ibid.

40 EBMWG, op. cit.

41 DiCenso et al, op. cit.

42 Popper, K. *Objective Knowledge: An Evolutionary Approach*, Oxford: Clarendon Press, 1979, p.261

43 Derrida, J. Différance. In J. Derrida *Margins of Philosophy*, New York: Harvester Wheatsheaf, 1982

44 Sim, S. *The Icon Critical Dictionary of Postmodern Thought*, Cambridge: Icon Books, 1998

45 Spivak, G.C. Translator's Preface. In J. Derrida *Of Grammatology*, Ballimore: The Johns Hopkins University Press, 1976, p.xvii

46 Derrida, 1976, op. cit., p.61

47 Ibid.

48 Lyotard, op. cit.

49 Ibid., p.142

ogy, London: Sage, 2000, p.154

8 Ibid., p.154

9 Bohm, D. *Wholeness and the Implicate Order*, London: Routledge, 1980

10 Fox, op. cit., p.179

11 Hebdige, D. Postmodernism and 'Politics' of style. In F. Frascina and J. Harris (eds) *Art in modern culture. An anthology of critical texts*, London: Phaidon, 1992, Ch32

12 Lodge, op. cit., p.193

13 Ibid., p.194

14 Department of Health *Making a Difference*, London: DoH, 1999

15 Bentz, V.M. and Shapiro, J.J. *Mindful Inquiry in Social Research*, California: Sage, 1998, p.31, emphasis in original

16 Fee, D. *Pathology and the Postmodern. Mental Illness as Discourse and Experience*, London: Sage, 2000

A response to Gary Rolfe
Faking a difference: evidence-based nursing and the illusion of diversity

David R Thompson

Gary Rolfe in a recent discursive article on diversity and evidence-based nursing (EBN) criticises Kevin Gournay, Nicky Cullum and me amongst others. He identifies us as being proponents of the dominant discourse of evidence-based practice and the randomised controlled trial (RCT). By association, therefore, we have 'power, money and fame'. If only!

Rolfe's thesis is that behind a 'façade of diversity... lies a core value of convergent conformism that serves to constrain individuality and style creativity' in nursing. In his prosecution he seems to level two charges. The first, and main one, is that I have written a paper on EBN and, because I hold a position 'of power and influence in the dominant discourse', I therefore, 'have most to gain in perpetuating the discourse and most to lose by its demise'. The other charge appears to be that I am based in the same department as Nicky Cullum, 'which has close links with the DoH'.

I plead guilty to both counts, though there were mitigating circumstances, your Honour, that I should like to have taken into account before being sentenced to eternal damnation!

The article to which Rolfe refers was an innocuous short paper commissioned by *Nursing Standard* to accompany a section devoted to EBN. I was asked to do this in my capacity as, then, Professor of Nursing Research at the DoH. Rolfe dwells in depth on the title of the paper, even to the extent of noting the absence of a question mark in the title. In my defence, I plead not guilty: I had no say in the title, which was provided by Nursing Standard after I had submitted the paper. Not that I make apologies for any of this, of course. However, I do challenge the assertion that I used 'outright denial' in the paper, and the assumption about what I was trying to convey in the paper. I was merely writing about what was in the brief of the commission, within the word limit I was given. It seemed eminently sensible to concentrate on research as I had been asked to talk about this, EBN and the NHS R&D Strategy. I resent the implication that I diminished the importance of 'clinical expertise'. As anyone who knows me or my work (with over 20 years experience in clinical nursing) will attest, I value highly this attribute.

Again, just for the record, I also value different research paradigms. Although I do not subscribe to the rather pejorative view that the RCT is the 'gold standard', I do think the RCT has an important role to play in clinical nursing research. I also happen to agree with Oakley[1] that divisions between qualitative and quantitative methods are unhelpful in the pursuit of useful knowledge.

Obviously, Rolfe is peddling his own views. He appears eager to establish his credentials by demonstrating that he is well read, with liberal reference to, for example, postmodernism, Derrida and deconstruction, as if there is universal agreement and acceptance of these. Terms such as 'postmodernism' are very ill defined[2]. In relation to Derrida, Wilson, for example, points out that 'It is not certain from Derrida's ornately obscurantist prose that he himself knows what he means'[3]. And, as Scruton notes, 'Deconstruction deconstructs itself, and disappears up its own behind, leaving only a disembodied smile and a faint smell of sulphur'[4].

Evidence-based nursing is an attempt to improve clinical practice and thus patient care. It is about solving clinical problems and it acknowledges that intuition and unsystematic clinical experience, for example, are insufficient as a basis for clinical decision making. Proponents of evidence-based practice also acknowledge that evidence alone is never sufficient to make a clinical decision; values and preferences play an important role[5]. Evidence-based practice is about weighing up the benefits and risks for individual patients. Nurses should admit that they are likely to have been involved in delivering care that was not only sub-optimal but was on occasions harmful to patients. I am not arguing that evidence-based nursing is a panacea, but Rolfe and other critics offer no better alternative to improve patient care.

Rolfe has clearly spent a good deal of time and effort analysing my paper, though I think he reads too much into it. He conveys a touch of disappointment, perhaps even a tinge of bitterness. I suspect he's a bit of a conspiracy theorist at heart. I think he should get out more!

Notes

1   Oakley, A . *Experiments in Knowing*, London: Polity, 2000

2   Gibbons, M., Limoges, C., Nowotny, H., Schwartzmann, S., Scott, P., Trow, M. *The New Production of Knowledge*, London: Sage, 1994

3   Wilson, E.O. *Consilience. The Unity of Knowledge*, London: Abacus, 1998, p.43

4   Scruton, R. *Modern Philosophy*, London: Sinclair-Stevenson, 1994, pp.478-9

5   Guyatt, G., Haynes, B., Jaeschke, R., Cook, D., Greenhalgh, T., Meade, M., Green, L., Naylor, C.D., Wilson, M., McAlister, F., Richardson, W.S. Introduction: the philosophy of evidence-based medicine. In G. Guyatt & D. Rennie (eds) *Users' Guide to the Medical Literature. A Manual for Evidence-based Clinical Practice*, Chicago: AMA Press, 2002

Faking an argument: prejudice-based views and the illusion of scholarship

Roger Watson

Certain aspects of the evidence-based practice movement receive a well deserved swipe in Gary Rolfe's paper. Anyone who has read *Friends in low places* by James Willis[1] will appreciate, evidence pointing to the hallmarks of totalitarianism are contained in the way the present government is trying to ensure uniformity, even mediocrity, across the board in healthcare. However, the problem is due to the fact that the majority of healthcare operates within a totalitarian system: the UK National Health Service, which in turn, is a corner-stone of a socialised, even socialist, political system. However, the origins of evidence-based practice were genuine efforts to seek the best practice, based on available research evidence, in the face of ritualistic and often damaging practice[2]. It is a terrible cliché, but Rolfe would have us toss the baby out with the bath water and, in the process, has based his arguments on a wrong premise and made personal and unwarranted attacks on distinguish-ed figures in UK nursing. I will not patronise those figures by trying to defend them in detail: each is more than capable of doing so alone. However, the links made between individuals by Rolfe are coincidental at best and their supposed 'power and influence' is earned rather than awarded by the Department of Health and their colleagues in the profession.

Rolfe sees the current developments in healthcare as the result of the centralising and 'phobic' attitudes of Right leaning politicians, with the Left representing the decentralising and diversifying force in politics. Try telling that to the average former Eastern Block citizen, even after the fall of the Berlin Wall. I would also assert that Rolfe misses a chance in flagging up *Making a Difference*[3] as being intended to promote autonomous and questioning practitioners while it was clear from the outset that it was intended to end graduate nurse education as we knew it in pursuit of a quick fix for the current shortage of nurses and the non-evidence-based belief - perpetrated by the present government - that university educated nurses were not clinically competent. Ironically, one of the individuals berated by Rolfe has clearly nailed his colours to the mast regarding the current prob-lems in UK nurse education - more than once[4].

As has happened before, recently, Foucault and other post-modern philosophers are called upon to support the argument against systematic, quantitative research[5], as if quantitative research had nothing to offer nursing. Unfortunately for Rolfe, and others in his genre, they offer such arguments in the face of overwhelming evidence that science, in the Popperian sense[6], actually works. It is unnecessary to list the achievements of science; rather, it is sufficient to turn the table and ask - without in any way denigrating qualitative investigations - other than insights which could not be obtained by any other means, precisely what qualitative research has contributed to patient care? I am not saying that is has contributed nothing but the list will not be very long. However, methodological mudslinging will get us nowhere.

What will get us somewhere are arguments based on correct premises and which do not attack individuals. Unfortunately, while many including myself appreciate Rolfe's efforts to illuminate us about particular issues in nursing and his freedom to do so, he has not achieved it on this occasion.

Notes

1   Willis, J. *Friends in Low Places*, Oxford: Routledge, 2001
2   Sackett, D.L., Richardson, W.S., Rosenberg, W., Haynes, R.B. *Evidence-Based Medicine*, New York: Churchill Livingstone, 1997
3   Department of Health *Making a Difference*, London: Department of Health, 1999
4   Thompson, D.R., Watson, R. Academic nursing – what is happening to it and where is it going?, *Journal of Advanced Nursing*, 2001, 36: 1-2; Watson, R., Thompson, D.R. Recent developments in UK nurse education: horses for courses or courses for horses? *Journal of Advanced Nursing*, 2000, 32: 1041-1042
5   Paley, J. An archaeology of caring knowledge, *Journal of Advanced Nursing*, 2001, 36: 188-198
6   Popper, K . *Conjectures and Refutations: the Growth of Scientific Knowledge*, New York: Harper and Row, 1965

A response to Thompson and Watson

Gary Rolfe

I welcome the opportunity to respond to some of the
points made by Thompson and Watson, since I believe that
they both misunderstand and misrepresent the basic
premise of my paper. Since Watson's fundamental charge
against me is that I base my arguments on a wrong
premise, it is important that I attempt to show that it
is he and not me who is confused over my premise. Watson
and Thompson both offer essentially the same critique, so
I hope that they will forgive me for considering their
papers together.

I will begin with what I believe to be their most
unfounded and potentially damaging point. Watson claims
that I made 'personal and unwarranted attacks on
distinguished figures in UK nursing', whilst Thompson
adds that I 'criticise Kevin Gournay, Nicky Cullum and me
amongst others'. I have looked long and hard at what I
wrote, and as far as I am aware, I make no personal
attacks (warranted or otherwise) and criticise no one,
although I do attack and critique views advocated by a
number of 'distinguished figures' (not my terminology!).
Thompson, at least, is aware that the only personal
reference I make to him is that he holds a position 'of
power and influence in the dominant discourse' and that
he has 'close links with the DoH'. Thus, whilst Watson
points out that these 'distinguished figures in UK
nursing' (including Thompson) are 'more than capable of
defending themselves'from my 'personal and unwarranted
attacks', Thompson is happy to 'plead guilty to both
counts', albeit with mitigating circumstances.

I have rather laboured this point because nursing as
an academic discourse appears to have a longstanding
problem with critique, particularly when that critique
(as in this case) is founded in a discipline outside
nursing, and (as in this case again) where it questions
the views of 'distinguished figures'. Since my original
paper was arguing that part of the brief of the dominant
discourse in nursing is to maintain discipline (in both
senses of the word) power and control, perhaps I should
not be surprised.

Watson continues with what can only be described as a
willful misreading of my paper. Thus:

> Rolfe sees the current developments in healthcare as
> the result of the centralising and 'phobic' attitudes
> of Right leaning politicians, with the Left represent-
> ing the decentralising and diversifying force in
> politics. Try telling that to the average former
> Eastern Block citizen ...

What I actually said was that those in power face a
conflict between espousing a philosophy of diversity and
attempting to manage and control a diverse group of
empowered individuals. My point was that whereas 'Right
leaning' politicians and managers openly acknowledge this
problem, the political Left takes a more underhand
approach by outwardly acknowledging libertarian views
whilst secretly acting to counter them. And Watson
unwittingly provides an ideal example of my point in the
Eastern Block citizen, since Stalinism outwardly
proclaimed to be socialist and even democratic (witness
the former Eastern Bloc 'German Democratic Republic')
whilst actually repressing all forms of dissent and
individuality. I suspect, then, that if I *did* try telling
it to the average former Eastern Block citizen, she would
understand my point better than Watson appears to.

Both Thompson and Watson also miss the point in a far
broader and more general way. Each sees my paper as an
attack on evidence-based practice (EBP) and quantitative
research, so perhaps I might restate its basic premise
here. My paper was concerned with the way in which the
dominant discourse (which in nursing I take to be the
Government sponsored discourse of EBP) *appears* to promote
diversity whilst *at the same time* acting to close it
down. All this is spelt out quite clearly in the
abstract. My point in relation to EBP was not that it is
bad or ineffective, but that it *appears* to encourage and
accept a wide range of different forms of evidence as of
equal worth, whereas its hidden agenda is to promote a
strict hierarchy with the RCT at the top. Again, my point
is not that the RCT is bad or ineffective, but that a
certain deceit is involved in the way that it is presented within the framework of EBP. I therefore attempted to
'deconstruct' the discourse of EBP by pointing out these
inconsistencies in the work of Watson's 'distinguished
figures', which often exist side-by-side in the same
text.

Watson is therefore clearly missing the point (and the
premise) when he accuses me of arguing against 'systematic quantitative research' in particular and science in
general. Similarly, Thompson suggests that I am promoting

an unhelpful division between qualitative and quantitative research, whereas I am not concerned to promote or
denigrate either. What I actually said was that whilst
EBP appears to be advocating a diverse approach to
research design, this belies 'a barely disguised contempt
for methodologies from competing discourses as "weaker
forms of evidence"'.

In my original paper, I cited Kevin Gournay in support
of this 'barely disguised contempt', but Watson's
response to my paper will do just as well. Thus:

> Without in any way denigrating qualitative investiga-
> tions ... precisely what [has] qualitative research
> contributed to patient care? I am not saying that it
> has contributed nothing, but the list would not be
> very long.

And just to doubly reassure us that he is not 'in any way
denigrating qualitative investigations', he continues:
'however, methodological mudslinging will get us
nowhere'. Quite.

And so, with a weary inevitability, to postmodernism,
always considered fair game and a soft target, especially
by those who have themselves only read critiques of it.
Thompson tells us that 'Obviously, Rolfe is peddling his
own views. He appears eager to establish his credentials
by demonstrating that he is well read, with liberal
references to, for example, postmodernism, Derrida and
deconstruction'. First, whose views would he prefer that
I 'peddle'? Second, as to my 'liberal references to postmodernism', I use the term only once in the entire paper,
when I refer to the 'postmodern architect Charles
Jencks'. And third, as to Derrida and deconstruction, I
refer liberally to both, not in order to demonstrate that
I am well read, but because my entire argument is based
on Derrida's methodology of deconstruction. Incidently, I
am well-read in Derrida's work, but I fail to see why
this might be a problem. Would Thompson prefer that,
instead of using the original source material, I do as he
did and refer only to two rather dubious secondary and
highly biassed critiques of deconstruction? And while we
are on the subject of these secondary sources, I would
suggest that Thompson comes much closer to personal
attack than I ever do when he cites E.O. Wilson and Roger
Scruton in their rants (I'm afraid that this is the only
word that does justice to what they write) against
Derridian deconstruction. Thus, whilst Watson calls for
arguments 'which do not attack individuals', Derrida

seems to be fair game, possibly because he is not one of Watson's 'distinguished figures in nursing'.

However, Scruton's rant against deconstruction does, inadvertently, make a valid point. 'Deconstruction deconstructs itself' he helpfully points out, in the mistaken belief that he is making a devastating critique. Well, of course it does, and if Scruton understood what deconstruction was about, he would see that this strengthens its case rather than negating it. Why, after all, should deconstruction be exempt from its own method of critique? But can we say the same about EBP? Where are the RCTs and systematic reviews that provide the evidence for the effectiveness of EBP? Thompson says that I invoke deconstruction as if there is universal acceptance of it. I might level the same accusation at both Thompson and Watson in their (almost) unconditional acceptance of EBP. As Thompson argues, EBP is not a panacea, but it is the best we have. My question to Thompson would be: on what evidence is that assumption based?

Thompson concludes by advising me to get out more. I wish to conclude with the observation that it is nursing that needs to get out more. It needs to look beyond the same tired old authorities and the same tired old arguments (and, I might add, the same tired old rants against postmodernism). Part of my attempt at deconstructing EBP involved challenging the interminable binary oppositions such as quantitative:qualitative, Leftist:Rightist politics and evidence:experience. Perhaps Thompson and Watson have these (and other) dichotomies and oppositions so embedded in their psyche that they read into my deconstruction of them a tacit support for one 'side' over the other. And finally, if writers wish to critique deconstruction, then they should *critique* it (unfortunately, that entails rather a lot of reading of primary sources) rather than simply citing insults from other writers who probably have not read the primary sources either. I think that this is what Watson refers to in the title of his paper as 'prejudice-based views and the illusion of scholarship'.

Deconstruction 3

Analyse this

... the phallus is none other than the concept, yes, the concept in itself, the possibility of the concept, of the concept in itself. The phallus is the concept, you can't oppose it, any more than you can oppose a 'sexual theory'. Unless you do something different, you can only oppose to it another concept or another theory, a knowledge like another. Very little.[1]

The middle (of course)

Not for the first time in this book I have decided not to begin at the beginning, nor do I want to start at the end, but I have a curiosity for beginning somewhere in the middle and working outwards, simultaneously, towards the beginning and the end. Of course, you might say, it doesn't matter where you start; it is still the beginning for me, the reader. The writer may have begun the process of writing the chapter long before the first words were typed, but for the reader the chapter always begins with the opening sentence. Nevertheless the opening sentence of any dialogue is always a middle sentence in (a) further conversation(s). And so it seems that I have begun before I even started.

Let us begin, then, with a fragment of discourse between Carl Rogers (C) and 'Miss Tir' (S) from the middle of a therapeutic counselling session that is itself in the middle of a series of sessions.

From ninth interview

S: This morning I hung my coat out there instead of here in your office. I've told you I like you, and I was afraid if you helped me on with the coat, I might turn around and kiss you.

C: You thought those feelings of affection might *make* you kiss me unless you protected yourself from them.

S: Well another reason I left the coat out there is that I want to be dependent - but I want to show you I don't have to be dependent.

C: You both want to be, and to prove you don't have to be.

Towards end of interview

S: I've never told anyone they were the most wonderful person I've ever known, but I've told you that. It's not just sex. It's more than that.

C: You feel really very deeply attached to me.

From tenth interview - toward close of interview

S: I think emotionally I'm dying for sexual intercourse but I don't do anything about it....The thing I want is to have sexual intercourse with you. I don't dare ask you, 'cause I'm afraid you'd be nondirective.

C: You have this awful tension, and want so much to have relations with me.

S: *(Goes on in this vein. Finally)* Can't we do something about it? This tension is awful! Will you relieve the tension ...Can you give me a direct answer? I think it might help both of us.

C: *(Gently)* The answer would be no. I can understand how *desperately* you feel, but I would not be willing to do that.

S: *(Pause. Sigh of relief.)* I think that helps me. It's only when I'm upset that I'm like this. You have strength and it gives me strength'[2].

Discourse analysis

According to Travers[3] discourse analysis has become one of the fastest growing areas of work within the human sciences. The term 'discourse' itself is an umbrella term used for a variety of different approaches to language and is usually used in preference to 'language' as it goes beyond language to sets of organised meanings (which can include images as well as words) on a given theme. Thus the term discourse 'has been used to emphasise the organised way in which meanings cohere around an assumed central proposition, which gives them their value and significance'[4]. Here I am viewing language and its use as a form of social action, in which talk is seen as contradictory or varied, constructed by individuals in order to serve certain interests. Thus, rather than language being descriptive of the world, it is constitutive of the world, worthy of investigation because of its effects. Language, then, is used to 'do' things: to control; to create a good impression; to persuade; to accuse and to request[5]. Language represses certain phenomena and enhances others, and as Billig[6] notes, is simultaneously expressive and repressive. The aim of a discourse analysis which holds such a social constructionist philosophy is to demonstrate how wider social structures (macro structures) shape the actions and beliefs of individuals in particular situations (micro structures) and vice versa.

Social discourse

Drawing upon the philosophical basis of social constructionism, discourse analysis provides not only an alternative way of viewing the use of clinical material in professional research/writing but also offers the possibility of broadening out a discussion, allowing for epistemological pluralism. Although it is difficult to define social constructionism, it differs from positivistic psychology in a number of ways. The social constructionist critique of positivism is based on the fact that it adopts a completely different ontological position in regard to the phenomena of the world. For example, in direct contrast to the positivistic belief that there is a truth which is waiting to be discovered, social constructionism takes the view that there is no such thing as 'objective' reality 'out there' in the world.

Social constructionism challenges the positivist notion of evidence-based medicine and clinical outcomes on the grounds that it treats such things as real, as opposed to being social constructions that have appeared in our discourses over time.

Gergen[7] argues for four fundamental assumptions in social constructionist work: that there is a radical doubt in the taken for granted world (this can be linked to the scepticism discussed in earlier chapters); that knowledge is viewed as historically, culturally and socially embedded (context bound); that knowledge is sustained by social processes and is not dependent upon empirical validity; and that explanations and descriptions of phenomena are constitutive of social action which serves to create and maintain some patterns to the exclusion of others (and as such can never be whole, true or objective). Social constructionism then challenges the notion of a grand theory, locating language as central to the way we view the world, and suggesting that reality and truth are socially constructed.

To say that there is no such thing as 'objective reality' is not to deny that there really is a world of things and people in the Newtonian sense. As Lomax cautions: 'It would be naive, I fear, to deny the existence of the Newtonian world, that world which is taken to be "out there", independent of the observer and consisting of a collection of identifiable things. Yet this world is only one story amongst others[8].

In this third and final deconstruction, I am going to (partially) analyse five stories, five worlds.

The first	The second	The third	The fourth	The fifth
world is the discourse of psycho-therapy, and in particular, the world of Rogerian client centred therapy.	world is the discourse of the taboo against sexual intercourse between client and therapist.	world is a small extract of spoken discourse between therapist Carl Rogers and one of his clients.	world is the discourse of EBP, that determines which therapies are considered to be most effective.	world is the discourse of discourse analysis itself, a discourse that is self-consciously examining itself.

These worlds, and my analysis of the discourses that constitute them, run parallel to each other, but they are not enclosed, not completely isolated. Sometimes these discourses intermingle and entwine, sometimes they borrow from one another. They are, however,

separate worlds, separate discourses.	separate worlds, separate discourses.	separate worlds, separate discourses.	separate worlds, separate discourses.	separate worlds, separate discourses.

You will notice that what follows is also itself a discourse, in which the voices of Freshwater (F) and Rolfe (R) (and several others) intermingle with those of Rogers (C) and his patient (S).

Inter-course analysis

F:　In 1992 at the Annual General Meeting of the British Association for Counselling (BAC), an amendment was made to the *Code of Ethics and Practice for Counsellors*. In summary, this amendment specified that it was not only unethical for counsellors to engage in sexual activity with their clients but that it was also equally unethical for counsellors to engage in sexual activity with their ex-clients for twelve weeks after the termination of the counselling relationship. I remember at the time wondering, with some amusement, how the 'expiry' date of the therapeutic relationship (twelve weeks) had been arrived at, and moreover, how this amendment would be enforced.

S: This morning I hung my coat out there instead of here in your office. I've told you I like you, and I was afraid if you helped me on with the coat, I might turn around and kiss you.

R: Some discourses are held to be self-evidently true. The most under-analysed discourse in the entire field of psychiatry, indeed, in all of health care, is the discourse of the ethics and pragmatics of the sexual relationship between therapist and client. Even the discourse of death, in the guise of euthanasia, is more open to exploration than the discourse of sex. The idea of the therapist killing the client is more acceptable to many people than the idea of sexual intercourse between them. The taboo surrounding sexual intercourse in/as therapy extends even to discussion and analysis of the taboo.

F: Over the last decade there have been many contentious debates and deliberations around this dictum, not least since the drive towards the professionalisation of both counselling and psychotherapy. The amendment, and subsequent additions, were introduced and passed on the advice of 'experts' in the field whom, it could be argued, relied on a purely subjective (and some might say emotional) response. Little 'hard' evidence existed to suggest that engaging in sexual activity with one's client (either during or after the conclusion of the therapeutic alliance) was harmful (to either the client or the therapist). It would seem that this powerful maxim, which was overwhelmingly voted in by BAC members, was therefore instated on the basis of subjective opinions and individual (assuming that there is such a thing) and collective moral consciousness. It is interesting to observe that a maxim, based almost entirely upon the evidence of 'expert' opinion, has been so widely acknowledged, even by those who question the value of such evidence.

A therapist writes: Erotic fantasies and desires need be no more detrimental to the analytic process than any other feelings such as jealousy, rivalry, hate, compassion, love, etc. I would suggest that it is not the existence or experience of these feelings that is problematic. Rather, they are for the therapist to scrutinize in self-analysis so they can be utilized in the analytic relationship in the interest of the patient. In my opinion, the hasty denial of repression of erotic drives is more likely to have a detrimental effect.[9]

C: You thought those feelings of affection might *make* you kiss me unless you protected yourself from them.

R: Who would conduct a randomised controlled trial on the therapeutic benefits of sleeping with clients?

Who would volunteer for such a study? How would it be single/double blinded? In the absence of a randomised controlled trial, what then would count as 'best' evidence? Patient preference? Who are the 'expert patients' in such cases? Patients who have already slept with their therapists? Those who have been spurned by their therapists? Or those who have turned down sexual advances from their therapists? It is difficult to see, then, what might count as evidence either for or against sexual intercourse within a therapeutic relationship. The very concept of 'thera-peutic' sexual intercourse stands permanently outside the discourse of evidence-based practice.

Psycho? Of course

F: So far I have suggested that discourse analysis can be beneficial in investigating the ideological implications of the language we use ordinarily. But what of the language that is used in discourses that are examining language and its inherent ideologies, for example psycho-therapy and counselling? These practices, which were once marginal and extraordinary, have only relatively recently become more main-stream. The English language is now replete with psychobabble, which it would seem has permeated our everyday existence. Psychotherapeutic discourse has, to a greater extent, become normalised; it infiltrates bookshops (witness the expanding bibliotherapy sections) and the media (the number of films which involve one of the main characters being in analysis has increased, along with the penchant for self-psychologising, as, for example, in the television series Ally McBeal and The Sopranos).

Discourses of psychotherapy, then, are widespread and may be encountered not only in the form of media, fiction, and local gossip, but also in theoretical and psychological models of development. According to Bruna-Seu[10] psychoanalysis 'looks for explanations of people's actions inside the person through an inquiry into their uncon-scious minds and their intrapsychic conflicts'. The patient, being made aware of her unconscious motivations, is enabled to see her unwitting repetitions in action through the analytic process, in the hope that she may replace the compulsion to repeat with a greater degree of con-scious choice. This view has been heavily criticised in recent years; Michel Foucault[11] in particular has strongly contested the existence of anything deep inside us that can be 'uncovered through recourse to experts (psychoanalysts, psychologists) whose knowledge provides privileged access to the person's self'.

R: Are all readings, all discourse analyses, equally valid? Or are some more socially accepted/acceptable

than others? And what does this mean? If all discourses are socially constructed, does this imply
some sort of democratic process, or are constructs
approved and validated by 'experts' appointed by the
very discourses that they are endorsing?

F: For Foucault, psychoanalysis is a powerful, ideologically driven confessional practice, one that normalizes oppressive social norms and
perpetuates the oppressive status quo, whilst simultaneously pathologis-
ing difference. R.D. Laing[12] provides a stark example in this discourse
between a consultant and a patient.

Consultant: and what is your complaint, apart from your acne, which we can
all see?

Patient: I'm afraid people are looking at me in the street

Consultant: you are afraid they know you masturbate

Patient: (His white face turned scarlet, and his red pimples went white)
yes

Consultant: how often do you masturbate?

Patient: two or three times a week

R: Discourse analysis challenges the authority of the
expert writer (and, indeed, the expert Writer, the
practitioner) and replaces it with the authority of
the expert reader. In some ways, discourse analysis
has a similar agenda to evidence-based practice,
although discourse analysts would claim that they do
not wish to replace one authority with another, but
to challenge the *very idea* of an authoritative reading. The question remains, however, of the authority
by which the claim to reject authority is made. In
other words, why should we believe the discourse
analyst when she tells us that all discourses are
social constructs? The only circumstances under which
we could take such a claim seriously is if the discourse of discourse analysis is somehow different
from the discourses that it is claiming to analyse;
if, in effect, discourse analysis is a *meta-
discourse*.

But why stop at social constructionism? Psychotherapy also makes a claim to be a meta-discourse in
the way that it attempts to analyse discourses of
normality and deviance. In its invocation of the
construct of the unconscious, it claims to have
access to discourses that are unavailable to other
methods of analysis. Similarly, evidence-based practice is clearly a meta-discourse (or what Lyotard
would call a metanarrative) in its claim that the discourse of science is elevated above, and can account

for, all competing discourses.

But we have seen that discourse analysis would wish to distance itself from evidence-based practice. If they are both meta-discourses, then they are employing the term 'meta-' in different ways. *Meta:* from the Greek, meaning 'of a higher or second order'[13]. Evidence-based practice regards itself as a higher order discourse, that is, as a discourse *above* or *superior to* other discourses of practice. Discourse analysis, on the other hand, regards itself as a second order discourse, that is, as a discourse *about* discourse. The discourse of discourse analysis is not claiming to be superior to other discourses in the sense of being more true, but rather to being the discourse by which other discourses can assess their own truth-claims. Each, in its own way, is concerned with power and authority.

F: Foucauldian discourse analysis is an analysis of power, and the complex ways that power and ideology permeate society and social practices. His detailed analyses of psychotherapeutic (and other) practices demonstrate how discourses stimulate the shift from external coercion to internal regulation through the person exercising surveillance upon themselves. This deep concern with the power imbalance in therapy has produced, of late, a very important shift in psychotherapy to narrative and discourse. In these approaches it is argued that psychoanalysis can be curative through attuning the patient to the analytic process itself, including its relativistic and fictional nature. This it to say that whilst therapy is helping the patient to explore the discourses by which they are named and constituted, it is also important to signify to the patient that the therapy itself is yet another discourse that the patients runs the risk of being constituted, named and motivated by. And, indeed, one that is no better or worse, true or false, right or wrong, than the guiding fictions that they currently cling to. What then is the business of psychotherapy?

R: From a Foucauldian perspective, the 'no sex' policy can be seen as a means for individual therapists to demonstrate their claim to be professionals through regulating their own desire. Since many men claim that sexual desire is the most difficult to control, such sexual self-regulation is a powerful symbol of professionalism. The professional therefore has much to gain by appearing to stand above the 'messy' world of sex.

Laing: I was sitting in, as a young psychiatrist, on a session of analytic group therapy, run by a psychoanalytically orientated psychiatrist who had not had, however, the benefit of a full psychoanalytic training. We sat in a circle in upright chairs with no sidearms for an hour and twenty minutes once a week. No smoking.

The patients were four men and four women, strangers to each other, and to him. All had met for the first time in the context of the group.

The psychiatrist's technique was to confine himself to transference interpretations. He restricted his movements, expressions and gestures to a minimum, in order to give away as little as possible of the counter-transference.

At one point, he interpreted an argument about politics between two of the men as an attempt to display and to conceal their desire to masturbate, mutually, and with him.

One of them turned to the psychiatrist, and asked:

'Doctor, do you masturbate?'

The psychiatrist was a decent chap. He was not a psychoanalyst, but he was a seasoned psychiatrist. He wriggled. Everyone watched and waited. He smiled.

'I've never known anyone who hasn't.'

The tension relaxed. He had blown it. Do you see why?[14]

R: *The tension relaxed. He had blown it...*

F: Whatever the business of psychotherapy and counselling, it is now a more widely accepted social practice, and certainly its increasing desire for professionalisation indicates a willingness to be part of a broader discourse of regulation and inclusion (hence such organisations as the British Association for Counselling and Psychotherapy, and the United Kingdom Council for Psychotherapy). Nevertheless, mental illness still carries with it a discourse of stigma. Any dominant discourse produces subject positions, subject positions being places in the discourse which carry certain rights to speak and specifications for what may be spoken[15]. In addition, subject positions determine the self at any given moment, some subject positions being favoured over others because they serve the positive development of our sense of self and self-esteem. As these are always relative and contextual, there will always be contradictions within speech[16]. Hence, depending upon whether I am the regulated or the regulator in any given moment, my subject position might change. Psychotherapists, at least, are simultaneously both regulators and regulated.

S: Well another reason I left the coat out there is that I want to be dependent - but I want to show you I don't have to be dependent.

C: You both want to be, and to prove you don't have to be.

R: *In a similar way, we might perhaps see the discourse of evidence-based practice as self-regulation by the practitioner of the desire to demonstrate expertise or to follow her intuition. Since intuition is an unconscious (or, at best, a subconscious) urge to* demonstrate her expertise through practising in a certain way, then the ability to regulate and suppress this desire is likewise seen as a potent symbol of professionalism. The contradiction is, however, rather obvious. The evidence-based practitioner demonstrates her professionalism by suppressing the most overt and obvious symbol of that very professionalism; she becomes an expert by suppressing her expertise. The evidence-based practitioner needs to demonstrate her professional dependence on scientific evidence, but wishes also to show that she does not have to be dependent on it.

We can see this contradiction very clearly in the literature of evidence-based practice, for example, in *Deconstruction 1*, where expertise is *at the same time* both exalted as an essential aspect of practice, and demeaned as of lesser importance to practice based on evidence from research. Expertise is a position of both strength *and* weakness; the evidence-based practitioner is both the regulator of, and is regulated by, the evidence.

Social Intercourse

A therapist writes: While we may be content for the moment to agree that sexual relations between psychotherapist and patient are unethical, in California, according to Susie Orbach, licensed psychotherapists are *required* to hand to every patient a leaflet which boldly states, 'Sex is always wrong' The mind boggles at the effect this must have on the person entering the therapy, at the messages it is sending out.[17]

Freud: The only unnatural sexual behaviour is none at all.

R: On what is this self-evident ethical discourse that 'sex is always wrong' based? Why is it considered ethical to administer electric shocks to patients against their will in order to induce a seizure, but not to sleep with them? Is it something to do with the therapist not exploiting his (and it usually is a 'he') power over his client when she (and it usually is a 'she') is in a vulnerable state? And is not the client who expresses a wish to sleep with her therapist *always* in a vulnerable state? Is not the expressed desire to sleep with her therapist *proof in itself* that the patient is not 'in her right mind'? Have we not pathologised this desire by labelling it as 'transference'?

F: In his account of client centred psychotherapy, Carl Rogers[18] provides brief excerpts of work with a client he refers to as Miss Tir. He writes of the

client: 'she (Miss Tir) is a person so deeply disturbed that she would
probably have been diagnosed as psychotic in terms of an external
evaluation'. He continues by adding that attitudes such as hers might
be more frequently found in a 'psychiatric ward or a state hospital' (210).
I am not sure how Rogers arrives at this conclusion, although I have to
assume that is not based purely on Miss Tir's sexual desire for her therapist. Interestingly, however, this statement precedes an excerpt that
specifically refers to Miss Tir's sexual tension.

R: Whose sexual tension? Miss Tir? Mister? Whatever was
Rogers thinking when he came up with this pseudonym?

S: I've never told anyone they were the most wonderful person I've
ever known, but I've told you that. It's not just sex. It's more than
that.

C: You feel really very deeply attached to me.

R: Rogers clearly does not take this comment at face
value, and chooses to respond to it as a manifestation of the patient's underlying pathology, referring
to it as 'an extreme example' of transference[19]. He
therefore deliberately ignores the enormous compliment that the client is paying him and responds with
a non-judgmental and emotionally neutral comment.
However, in not responding to the compliment, he is
indicating its lack of validity, suggesting that it
is insincere, or at least that it is being made
whilst the client was in some way 'not in her right
mind'. To what extent, then, is Rogers' attempt at
being non-judgmental itself a judgmental act?

F: Although it is some fifty years since the first edition of this text, sexuality
(and, in particular, female sexuality) still remains a taboo subject within
society. As with all taboos (which in themselves may not be particularly
alluring, but certainly become more appealing once they are
constructed as taboos), it holds a deep fascination and mystery[20].
Hence, it becomes something that not only has multiple discourses
associated with it, but is also itself associated with extremely powerful
discourses. And as Focault[21] reminds us, where there is power there is
resistance. One might argue that there is no better place to explore
resistance, taboo and power than in psychotherapy. Yet, it is psychotherapy that has created at least one of the taboos around sexual
activity that it seeks to deconstruct.

A therapist writes: There are many reasons why analysis and a love relationship between the same partners is not only inappropriate but can do
harm to both. In the first place, collective unconsciousness in our society
and in our profession condemns a concrete love relationship between
analyst and analysand. Now an analyst may feel this to be an outdated

superego attitude, and believe that individuation actually means not to identify with collective moral standards but to adapt them to genuine situations in real life. On this basis he might make a personal decision to act out the emotional attraction. But at the same time he and his analysand have to live in our society, and the decision to be both analyst and lover would inevitably put a lot of strain on their relationship. The collective disapproval is so great that both would have to keep absolute secrecy.[22]

F: Psychotherapy is an enabling process, one which is designed to help the client grow to greater maturity through learning to take responsibility and to make decisions for themselves.

A therapist writes: A really satisfying sexual relationship can indeed be most valuable and more rewarding than any amount of therapy.[23]

A patient writes to his therapist: To get back to you and me. The horrible thing is that I understand, from things you said and from my reading, the explanation for my feelings for you - that they're transference feelings, a way of reliving the past, etc. I understand fully; I'm even, in some sense, willing to accept the explanation. I tell myself everyday, in a half-humorous, civilised tone: 'Be sensible there, fellow - it isn't *her* you have these feelings for,' and I quote old Freud to myself, and old whoever-else-it-was I read, and I pat myself on the back for being superior to those pathetic housewives you hear about who, not understanding a thing about transference, imagine themselves to be in love with their doctors. Doesn't do a bit of good, Wanda. In my heart I am those house-wives.[24]

R: Freud's first encounter with transference came vicar-iously through the work of his colleague, Joseph Breuer. Breuer claimed to have been taken completely by surprise during his psychoanalysis of Anna O, although a more astute Freudian would perhaps have had his suspicions aroused by Anna's description of her sessions with Breuer as 'chimney sweeping'. Freud's translator, James Strachey, recounts how 'when the treatment had apparently reached a success-ful end, the patient suddenly made manifest to Breuer the presence of a strong unanalysed positive trans-ference of an unmistakably sexual nature. It was this occurrence, Freud believed, that caused Breuer to hold back the publication of the case history for so many years'.[25] Elsewhere, Ernest Jones recounts how Breuer 'fled the house in a cold sweat. The next day he and his wife left for Venice to spend a second honeymoon, which resulted in the conception of a daughter'.[26]

A patient writes to his therapist: And who's to say we aren't right, we house-wives? Who's to say I don't, or don't 'really', love that sympathetic, quietly

attentive young woman with the soulful eyes and the dandy legs. However you try to account for it, it's you I love. No reason I couldn't, no
reason I shouldn't. Except that maybe you don't love me - but what kind
of reason is that? And if you don't, why won't you come right out and say
so? Then I'd know where I stood. Then I'd know what I was up against.
Then I could go about making myself absolutely irresistible. All I want is
the same chance you'd give to any one of a hundred other men.[27]

R: For Freud, transference can be safely ignored until
it begins to interfere with treatment, at which point
it should be addressed head-on and thereby transformed into a therapeutic tool. For Rogers, however, the
interpretation of transference hinders rather than
helps therapy.

Freud: It is out of the question for us to yield to the patient's demands deriving
from the transference; it would be absurd for us to reject them in an
unfriendly, still more in an indignant, manner. We overcome the transference by pointing out to the patient that his feelings do not arise from
the present situation and do not apply to the person of the doctor, but
that they are repeating something that happened to him earlier.... By that
means the transference, which, whether affectionate or hostile, seemed
in every case to constitute the greatest threat to the treatment, becomes
its best tool, by whose help the most secret compartments of mental life
can be opened.[28]

Rogers: To me it seems clear that the most effective way of dealing with *all*
feelings directed toward the therapist is through the creation of a therapeutic relationship that fulfills the conditions set forth in client-centred
theory. To deal with transference feelings as a very special part of
therapy, making their handling at the very core of therapy, is to my mind
a grave mistake. Such an approach fosters dependency and lengthens
therapy. It creates a whole new problem, the only purpose of which
appears to be the intellectual satisfaction of the therapist - showing the
elaborateness of his or her expertise. I deplore it.[29]

A patient writes to his therapist: So fuck transference. Transference is the
story you tell yourself to make a dirty business sound clean. Transference is your way of distorting my feelings. It's your way of avoiding
me. Of pretending I don't exist. Worse yet, of pretending *you* don't exist.
It's your way of living with what you do in case something goes wrong.[30]

F: Haule points out that Eros is often misunderstood as sexual desire. He
argues that 'the "erotic" refers to the energy of an interpersonal field
when a sense of *we-ness* comes forcefully to presence and that the
sexual involves an impulse to embody that *we-ness* in a genital
manner[31]. Love, he suggests, requires us to maintain a distance amid
our union, a distance that retains our I-ness and you-ness.

S: I think emotionally I'm dying for sexual intercourse but I don't do anything about it ... The thing I want is to have sexual intercourse with you. I don't dare ask you, 'cause I'm afraid you'd be nondirective.

R: Perhaps we have to ask ourselves at this point who has the most insight in this encounter and who is being most genuine about their feelings. Rogers' assumption is that he is more in touch with the feelings of his client than she is herself; that she thinks that she wishes to sleep with him, whereas she really wishes to sleep with her father. She is therefore 'not in her right mind', and so any sexual contact would take advantage of her vulnerable state. Of course, if Rogers was to take a (preferably sane) woman to dinner, buy her several drinks and then accept her offer of sexual intercourse, few people would consider his behaviour morally reprehensible, despite the fact that the woman could be said to be in a vulnerable state through taking a drug that has the specific effect of lowering sexual inhibitions.

F: We can see, then, that it is easy to confuse the seductive pull to an incestuous merger with that of a deep longing for the divine. In relation to the 'madness' of sexual acting out, Schwartz-Salant warns 'If repression occurs rather than transformation, we engender a shadow side to the analysis'[32] and 'the god Dionysus takes a toll from those who deny him'[33]. Donleavy critiques Rutter's well-known account in *Sex and the Forbidden Zone* of how he withdrew from an attempted seduction by his patient by asking her to return to her chair. Donleavy claims that failure to stay with the erotic tension by avoidance or acting out, disallows the potential for a healing image or experience to occur:

A therapist writes: With either choice the unconscious psychic part that was experienced through the desire or the fear stay still unconscious. If the tension can be held and the psychic part made conscious in each person, the couple will feel not the overwhelming need for physical merger but a psychic resonance between them. This resonance will also be experienced as a new intrapsychic wholeness.[34]

F: The key to her statement is 'If the tension can be held'.

C: You have this awful tension, and want so much to have relations with me.

R: A non-answer to a non-question. *If the tension can be held*, and not identified as transference (Freud), not ignored in the hope that it will go away (Rogers) and not actively avoided (Breuer). It would appear that the discourse of psychotherapy is not ethically equipped to hold on to the tension. The therapist is

unwilling (or unable) to sustain a situation in which
he is the object of desire.

Professional Intercourse

F: It is far from obvious that professionalism will result in better standards of
       psychotherapeutic work. Psychotherapy, unlike medicine or law, cannot
       easily espouse the objective model of the person. Rather, psychothera-
       pists are engaged in a particular type of conversation with those they
       see in an attempt to understand the difficulties in their lives. A conversa-
       tion within the context of a therapeutic hour can appear absurd once
       translated into a different context, even that of professional supervision,
       making external regulation of psychotherapeutic practices very prob-
       lematic.

       Although Foucault was writing some time ago, it is interesting to review
       his analyses in the context of the contemporary developments in clinical
       supervision, not only in psychotherapeutic practices but also across all
       health related disciplines. The discourse surrounding clinical supervision
       normally includes something around professional development, support
       and education for the supervisee, and quality control measures.
       Although the concept of an internal supervisor is not new (see for
       example Casement's work[35]) little is written regarding the development
       of an internal regulator from the perspective of Foucauldian discourse
       analysis. It seems that when agreeing to abide by the various (but
       convergent) Codes of Ethics for Counselling and Psychotherapy, what
       therapists are signing up to is a covenant about accepting and abiding
       by a discourse that normalises a profession which in turn normalises
       discourses of development, behaviour, mental health, and so on. Within
       a social constructionist or discursive framework, the reality of mental
       health problems may appear to be denied; after all, they are a
       construct of society, a construct that is normalised and internalised by
       therapeutic discourse itself. Thus madness, neurosis, schizophrenia, can
       all be conceptualised merely as social labels or categories. This is not
       too far away from the visionary work of R.D. Laing, who gives this
       example of the social construction of depression (and its cure!).

Laing: One enthusiast [of ECT] in London goes around publicly giving figures
       of 85 per cent remission of symptoms in electric shock treatment for
       involutional depression, and comparable figures for all sorts of other
       conditions, including children who don't want to have anything to do with
       other people, seventeen-year-old hysterics, and so on. He gets 'very
       good results' so far as I hear. He comes around in the morning, does the
       ward rounds. 'How are you today? Better or worse?' And if you don't say
       you're better, you get another course of electric shock treatment. Most
       people say they are better, and most of them do not report back to the
       out-patient department.[36]

S: (*Goes on in this vein. Finally*) Can't we do something about it? This tension is awful! Will you relieve the tension... Can you give me a direct answer? I think it might help both of us.

C: (*Gently*) The answer would be no. I can understand how *desperately* you feel, but I would not be willing to do that.

R: 'The answer *would be* no'. Hardly a direct answer. Why the conditional case? Why not 'The answer *is* no'? Or simply: 'No'? And similarly: 'I *would not* be willing to do that'. Why not: 'I *am not* willing to do that'? Or: 'I *will not* do that'? Or even: 'I *don't want* to do that'? Always the possibility that Rogers does want to do it, but that his 'ethical code' prevents him. And, as we shall see, this is how his response appears to be interpreted by the client.

F: Speaking about himself in the future tense, Rogers manages to disassociate, observing himself (no doubt from the moral high ground) rather than experiencing himself and his visceral reaction to Miss Tir.

A therapist writes: It may on the other hand be terribly irritating and annoying to be the victim of so many unwanted demands. Or it may be a satisfaction to the analyst's masculine vanity that women fall in love with him so intensely.[37]

F: So questions may be asked regarding whose interests are served by maintaining the discourse of stigma around mental illness: how and who does it serve to control the psychotherapy profession, and whom and what is it attempting to persuade about psychotherapy? Certainly psychotherapy benefits from (and indeed perpetuates and is reliant upon) the maintenance of the dominant discourse which defines 'normal' and 'acceptable' behaviour in opposition to 'pathological' and 'intolerable' behaviour. But as Ussher notes, one of the main problems with arguing that madness exists entirely at a discursive level and adopting such a radical social constructionist perspective is that 'we are implicitly denying the influence of biology or genetics, and diminishing the meaning ascribed to the body in general'[38]. Ussher, it would appear, is missing the point. The willingness to adopt a meta perspective toward the discursive prescriptions which regulate our practices might serve to at least 'mediate against unreflective and unwittingly iatrogenic practice'[39].

S: (*Pause. Sigh of relief.*) I think that helps me. It's only when I'm upset that I'm like this. You have strength and it gives me strength

R: 'You have strength and it gives me strength'. Rogers picks up on the second part of the client's statement: '... it gives me strength'. A successful therapeutic intervention, then. But what of the first

part: 'You have strength...'? Not: 'Oh well, you're
obviously not interested in a sexual relationship
with me', but: 'You appear to be interested but you
have the strength to resist'. To what extent is
Rogers' non-directive approach simply leading the
client on, maintaining her hope of a sexual relationship with him if and when his 'strength' fails?

Psycho-course

F: Psychoanalysis and discourse analysis enjoy some convergence of
ideas in that they both provide the opportunity to examine factors which
militate against change at the 'dynamic interplay between resistance to
power and resistance to change'[40]. However, as Hollway[41] points out,
psychoanalysis explores resistance to change at an intrapsychic level,
whilst discourse analysis examines the meanings and values attached to
a person's practices. Harper[42] notes that discourse analysis is extremely
useful when examining such phenomena as psychiatric categories,
which he says 'are produced almost entirely in language' (348). A
number of writers concur on this, observing that the discursive
examination of these psychiatric categories shifts them from being
merely an explanatory resource to regarding them as a topic to be
explored. One example of such a discursive examination is that of
Billig[43], who analysed the psychoanalytic text of Freud, and in particular,
Freud's notion of repression. Indeed, many social constructionists use
concepts from Freud, illustrating the attractions of psychoanalysis for
critical theorists[44].

R: The discourse of evidence-based practice makes a
similar claim to challenge resistance to change: it
is a 'new paradigm' intended to shake the practitioner out of her habitual and outdated mode of
practice. Although Phillips[45] argues that EBP challenges the 'new folklores' of practice that is not
based on research, it is perhaps interesting to
explore the extent to which evidence-based practice
has itself become a 'new folklore'. Consider, if you
will, the following extract from a letter by Sarah
Goodband[46], a nurse with diabetes admitted to hospital
for elective surgery:

A patient writes: I have only been diagnosed with diabetes for a short time.
On the whole my control is good, but when normal conditions are
removed, everything goes a bit pear-shaped. I explained this on
admission and raised my concern that since I was having surgery to my
shoulder, I was not sure how I would manage my injections and blood
sugar measurements. The anaesthetist told me that research showed
that people with diabetes were much better at handling their own control

in hospital than health professionals, and as soon as I was tolerating fluids and diet I could manage my own control. This all seemed reasonable, as presumably there would be someone to advise me. Back on the ward after the operation, the nurse told me about the research that proved how much better I would feel if I took control of my diabetes care. I ventured that just for once, it would be nice not to think about it. When supper arrived, things got rather surreal. The nurse asked me why I had not taken my normal insulin. I told her it was a little difficult as I had a brachial plexus block to my right arm. I was reminded of the research, and asked how much insulin I wanted to give. Since my blood sugar was four and I had no intention of eating as I felt nauseated, I asked her what she thought. 'You're the expert – you decide', she replied. I erred on the side of caution and gave nothing. The situation continued. The nurses were happy to give the insulin but I had to decide the dosage. Each nurse I asked for advice referred me back to the famous research.

Critical Discourse Analysis

F: Critical discourse analysis is a sub-field of discourse analysis, and combines resources and ideas from linguistics with concepts from critical theory. Writers using critical discourse analysis focus on the relationship between language and ideology[47]. The pivotal argument is that language must be studied from a political perspective, and that 'researchers working in linguistics can help emancipate people from false ideas through revealing how language serves the needs of the economically powerful'[48]. Thus, critical discourse analysts usually examine texts which communicate either a covertly concealed or overtly explicit political message; that is to say that any piece of text or dialogue can be used to advance a political argument. What, then, is the message that psychotherapy wishes to communicate (intentionally or not)? Further, what is the covertly concealed or overtly political message that is communicated through the 'No Sex Please, We're Psychotherapists' maxim?

R: For Rogers, the therapeutic effect of therapy is for the patient to be heard in a respectful and non-judgemental manner. However, the interesting thing about non-directive therapy is that although Rogers claims to be responding at a deep level to the emotional content of the client's discourse, his responses are largely interchangeable. This can easily be demonstrated simply by reversing the order of the discourse; that is, by reading it backwards:

S: (*Goes on in this vein. Finally*) Can't we do something about it? This tension is awful! Will you relieve the tension.... Can you give me a direct answer? I think it might help both of us.

C: You have this awful tension, and want so much to have relations with me.

S: I think emotionally I'm dying for sexual intercourse but I don't do anything about it.... The thing I want is to have sexual intercourse with you. I don't dare ask you, 'cause I'm afraid you'd be nondirective.

C: You feel really very deeply attached to me.

S: I've never told anyone they were the most wonderful person I've ever known, but I've told you that. It's not just sex. It's more than that.

F: In the world of evidence-based practice, the practitioner is able to respond to specified problems using empirically tested algorithms. Thus, there need be no discourse at all; the psychotherapist need not be 'present' as such. Rather, he can employ the prescribed (rehearsed) responses for the 'hysterical woman', remaining passive and objective in the encounter. The hysterical woman, experiencing the absence of the therapist's flaccid penis as disrespect, works harder to manipulate him to erection.

Discursive Therapy

Foucault advocated a necessary problematisation of commonplace presuppositions concerning social life. In this sense, deconstruction can be thought of as a kind of 'setting at risk, a relaxation of control and of the enforcement of stability'[49].

If life is the practice, then discursive therapy might be considered the re(search) for an evidence-based existence. As Parker comments: 'Within a discursive approach, it is the role of the therapist to explicate, situate and trace the history of the various discourses that are mediating the sense that those people who are consulting us in therapy are making of their experience'[50]. Further, 'In a politics of listening, one is searching for the form of colonizing discourses hidden in the apparent transparency of personal accounts'[51].

I have previously illustrated the role of politics and disguised liberalism masquerading as tolerance and diversity (see *Deconstruction 2*). Exposing the inherent contradictions in this way is threatening to the dominant discourse because, as Louis Althusser observed in the 1970s, capitalism (and capitalism disguised as liberalism) will eventually self destruct due to internal contradictions in the system. Social constructionism allows for a better representation of 'human diversity in contrast to more normative positivistic accounts'[52].

This is the beginning...

In previous chapters I have focussed on alternative ways of investigating practice, of writing practice, and of deconstructing and (re)constructing practice. In doing so I have also explored, in some detail, the epistemology and ontology of truth, which from a positivistic viewpoint, can be discovered and revealed through improved research methods and a position of detached objectivity. Discussions that link clinical scenarios and case material (which mainly rely on alternative 'definitions' of truth) to the notion of evidence-based medicine raise serious doubts in the mind of the positivist. Indeed, many positivist writers conclude that, on the whole, the use of case material in clinical writing is of little value, since its approach to data collection and analysis is methodologically unsound. Hence, the discourse around professional clinical discourse.

This chapter considers another way of investigating clinical discourse, that of discourse analysis. According to Parker[53], the attention given to the pre-eminent term discourse typifies the influence of postmodernism on psychotherapy. The term 'discursive therapy' is now used to describe those therapies embracing a social constructionist perspective; further, it is a convenient term for therapies which utilise discourse-related concepts, such as deconstruction, text, conversation and narrative. Curt[54], however, points out that there are remarkably different discourses of discourse available for articulation in discursive therapy, all of which have quite different implications for practice. Lowe distinguishes between 'discourse' that is used pragmatically to portray an ongoing process of interaction and 'Discourses' used within the Foucauldian framework, the latter pertaining to the 'systematic and instutionalised ways of speaking/writing which form the objects of which they speak *and* conceal their role in doing so'[55]. Thus, whilst pragmatic postmodernists might focus more on staying with the client's frame of reference, seeking to influence linguistic patterns, critical and social postmodernists are more interested in bringing non-therapy discourses into the therapeutic work, believing that it is crucial to go beyond individual sites of language to the broader social and institutional analyses. Curt[56], for example, is critical of discursive therapy because of its tendency to focus on individual sites of text, as opposed to the broader context of textuality. As Parker[57] reminds us, there is more to textuality than text.

Dissent in the academy

According to Karl Marx, the purpose of intellectual inquiry was not simply to understand the world, but more importantly, to change it. Whilst Marxism is no longer influential within universities, the last forty years has seen a dramatic rise in the number of new social movements seeking to change the way our societies are organised. Hence, 'New developments in social theory, in the form of postmodern and post structuralist theory, have replaced Marxism as a way of thinking critically about the world....'[58]. Thus, whilst Althusser viewed Marxism as a science, the critical theorists see it as an emancipatory movement akin to psychoanalysis.

Postmodern and poststructuralist thought poses serious challenges to the epistemological foundations of both Marxism and critical theory, proposing a further way of being critical in the academy. This paradigmatic shift, away from assumptions that the external world can be apprehended accurately through the senses and via information processing systems, leads to the belief that it is impossible to view the world directly. This shift is often referred to as the shift from 'world to word'[59]. 'Knowledge is, therefore, seen not as something that a person *has* (or does not have), but as something that people *do* together'[60]. Social constructionism has adopted the principle that it is possible to identify different discourses embedded in language. It is not surprising, then, that discourse analysis has also taken a critical turn.

Inconclusion...

...*(this is not the end)*

Notes

1   Derrida, J. (1998) *Veils*, Stanford, California: Stanford University Press, 2001, p.85

2   Rogers, C.R. *Client Centered Therapy*, London: Constable, 1951, p.211

3   Travers, M. *Qualitative Research Through Case Studies*, London: Sage, 2001

4   Hollway, W. and Jefferson, T. *Doing Qualitative Research Differently*, London: Sage, 2000, p.14

5   Potter, J. and Wetherell, M. *Discourse and Social Psychology: Beyond Attitudes and Behaviour,* London: Sage, 1987

6   Billig, M. *Talking of the Royal Family,* London: Sage, 1999

7   Gergen, K.J. The social constructionist movement in modern psychology, *American Psychologist,* 1985, 40, 266-275

8   Lomax, Y. *Writing the Image: An adventure with Art and Theory,* London: I.B. Tauris, 2000

9   Mann, D. *Psychotherapy: An Erotic Relationship,* London: Routledge, 1997

10 Bruna-Seu, I. Change and Theoretical Frameworks. In I. Bruna-Seu & M. Colleen Heenan (eds) *Feminism and Psychotherapy,* London: Sage, 1998, p.204

11 Foucault, M. *The History of Sexuality. Vol. 1: An introduction,* Harmondsworth: Penguin, 1981, p.204

12 Laing, R.D. *The Facts of Life,* Harmondsworth: Penguin, 1976, p.85

13 The New Penguin English Dictionary, Harmondsworth: Penguin

14 Laing, R.D. *The Voice of Experience: Experience, Science and Psychiatry,* Harmondsworth: Penguin, 1982, p.53

15 Parker, I. Discursive Psychology. In D. Fox & I. Prilleltensky (eds) *Critical Psychology,* London: Sage, 1997

16 Potter & Wetherell, op. cit.

17 Gordon, P. *Therapy as Ethics,* London: Constable, 1999, p.36

18 Rogers, op. cit., p.210

19 Ibid., p.210

20 Jacoby, M. *The Analytic Encounter: Transference and Human Relationship,* Toronto: Inner City Books, 1984

21 Foucault, M. *Power/Knowledge: Selected Interviews and Other Writings, 1972-77,* Brighton: Harvester, 1980

22 Jacoby, op. cit., p.105

23 Ibid., p.112

24 Twiggs, J. *Transferences,* Fayetteville: University of Arkansas Press, 1987

25 Strachey, J. Footnote in S. Freud & J. Breuer (1895) *Studies on Hysteria,* Harmondsworth: Penguin Books, 1974, pp.95-6

26 Jones, E. *Sigmund Freud: Life and Work, Vol. 1,* London: The Hogarth Press, 1956, p.247

27 Twiggs, op. cit.
28 Freud, S. (1917) *Introductory Lectures on Psychoanalysis*, Harmondsworth: Penguin, 1974, p.496
29 Rogers, C. (1987) Reflection of feelings and transference. In H. Kirschenbaum & V.L. Henderson (eds) *The Carl Rogers Reader*, London: Constable, 1990, p.134
30 Twiggs, op. cit.
31 Haule, J. *The Love Cure, Therapy Erotic and Sexual*, Dallas: Spring, 1996, p.55
32 Schwartz-Salant, S. *The Mystery of Human Relationships: Alchemy and the Transformation of Self*, London: Routledge, 1998, p.2
33 Ibid., p.112
34 Donleavy, P. *Analysis and Erotic Energies in The Interactive Field In Analysis,* Illinois: Chiron, 1995, p.110
35 Casement, P. *On Learning from the Patient*, London: Routledge, 1985
36 Laing, R.D. *The Facts of Life*, op. cit., p.110
37 Jacoby, op. cit., p.109
38 Ussher, J. Women's madness: a material discursive intrapsychic approach. In D. Fee (ed) *Pathology and Postmodernism*, London: Sage, 2000, p.218
39 Parker, op. cit., p.36
40 Bruna-Seu, op. cit., p.206
41 Hollway, W. Gender difference and the production of subjectivity. In J. Henriques, W. Hollway, C. Urwin, C. Venn, V. Walkerdine (eds) *Changing the subject: Psychology, Social Regulation and Subjectivity,* London: Routledge, 1984
42 Harper, D.J. Discourse analysis and 'mental health'. *Journal of Mental Health*,1995, 4, 347-357
43 Billig, op. cit.
44 Bordieu, P. *Pascalian Meditations*, Cambridge: Polity Press, 2000
45 Phillips, R. The need for research-based midwifery practice. *British Journal of Midwifery*, 1994, 2, 7, 335-8
46 Goodband, S. Research is the new nursing ritual. *Nursing Times*, 2001, 97, 25, p.21

47 Fairclough, N. *New Labour, New Language*, London: Routledge, 2000

48 Travers, op. cit., p.122

49 Parker, op. cit., p.167

50 Ibid., p.120

51 Ibid., p.96

52 Harper, op. cit., p.349

53 Parker, op. cit.

54 Curt, B. *Textuality and Tectonics: Troubling Social and Psychological Science*, Buckingham: Open University Press, 1994

55 Lowe, R. *Family Therapy and the Uses of Postmodernism: From Revisionism to Descriptivism*, University of Queensland: PhD Dissertation, 1995, p.52

56 Curt, op. cit.

57 Parker, op. cit.

58 Travers, op. cit., p.100

59 See, for example, Holloway & Jefferson, op. cit., Travers, op. cit., Chapman, J. The Rhythm Model. In I. Bruna-Seu & M. Colleen Heenan (eds) *Feminism and Psychotherapy*, London: Sage, 1998

60 Burr *An introduction to Social Constructionism*, London: Routledge, 1995, p.8

Afterword

*'For there must not be a last
word - that's what I'd like to
say finally; the afterword is
not, that means ought not,
ought never to be a last word'
(Jacques Derrida - Afterw.rds,
or at least, less than a
letter about a letter less)*

Afterword 1

Rules for reading

I tried to work out ... what was in no way meant to be a system but rather a sort of strategic device, opening onto its own abyss, an enclosed, unenclosable, not wholly formalizable ensemble of rules for reading, interpretation and writing.[1]

Pas de méthode...

If you have read as far as this Afterword, you will probably have realised that the most fundamental problem of writing a book about deconstruction is that it is almost impossible to define quite what deconstruction is. As Wolfreys has pointed out, if deconstruction consists in challenging the authority of the 'is', then any statement that attempts to describe what deconstruction *is*, is itself open to being deconstructed.[2] This perhaps explains why Derrida is usually very reluctant to provide any authoritative statement about deconstruction. Thus:

> ... deconstruction doesn't consist in a set of theorems, axioms, tools, rules, techniques, methods.... there is no deconstruction, deconstruction has no specific object ...[3]

Similarly, elsewhere he claims that:

> ...deconstruction is neither an analysis nor a critique.... I would say the same about method. Deconstruction is not a method and cannot be transformed into one.... It must also be made clear that deconstruction is not even an act or an operation ...[4]

and even:

> I have never claimed to identify myself with what may be designated
> by this name [deconstruction]. It has always seemed strange to me, it
> has always left me cold. Moreover, I have never stopped having
> doubts about the very identity of what is referred to by such a nick-
> name.[5]

Clearly, we have a problem; a problem that I have tried to resolve in this
book by simply presenting some examples of deconstruction without
very much in the way of theoretical underpinning. If deconstruction is not
a method, not an act, not an operation; if it is not reducible to theorems,
axioms, tools, rules or techniques; then it cannot be taught, cannot be
passed on to others except by example.

But as McQuillan has observed, Derrida's assertion that deconstruction is not a method *('pas de méthode')* can be 'read' in a different way:
'The word *pas* in French means both 'not' and 'step', so this ambiguous
phrase can be translated as either "not a method" or "a methodological
step"'[6]. Thus, in keeping with his insistence that deconstruction cannot
be tied down to a single meaning, Derrida reveals that his early work
from the 1960s consisted *precisely* in an attempt to formulate such a
strategy or methodological step that he elsewhere claims to be impossible:

> During the years that followed, from about 1963 to 1967, I tried to
> work out - in particular in the three works published in 1967 - what
> was in no way meant to be a system but rather a sort of strategic
> device, opening onto its own abyss, an enclosed, unenclosable, not
> wholly formalizable ensemble of rules for reading, interpretation and
> writing.[7]

Not a system, then, but an *ensemble of rules* for reading, interpretation
and writing. It is not entirely clear what these rules for reading, interpretation and writing might be, but Spivak gives us some clues in her
'Translator's Preface' to *Of Grammatology*:

> To locate the promising marginal text, to disclose the undecidable
> moment, to pry it loose with the positive lever of the signifier; to

reverse the resident hierarchy, only to displace it; to dismantle in order to reconstitute what is always already inscribed. Deconstruction in a nutshell [8]

As well as the general descriptor of deconstruction as *to dismantle in order to reconstitute what is already described*, we can discern three clear strategies by which such a dismantling might be accomplished. *To locate the promising marginal text*, that is, to write of, in and at the margins. *To disclose the undecidable moment, to pry it loose with the positive lever of the signifier*, that is, to expose the practice of double coding (or what Spivak calls 'double-edged words'). *To reverse the resident hierarchy, only to displace it*, that is, to expose and challenge binary opposites in the text. Each of these three strategies will now be discussed (in reverse order).

Challenging binary opposites

I will begin, then, with perhaps Derrida's favourite strategy: that of exposing and challenging the way that binary opposites are used to maintain the dominant discourse. Derrida points out that Western logic is structured around a tension between binary pairs such as rational:irrational, progress-ive:backward, scientific:mystical, masculine:feminine, reason:superstition, and so on. However, these binary pairs are not simply regarded as oppo-sites, as equal but complementary; rather, the first term in each pair is seen as superior to, or privileged over, the second. Furthermore, this unequal privileging of the rational over the irrational, of the scientific over the mystical, of the masculine over the feminine, what Derrida refers to as 'logocentrism', is so ingrained in Western culture from the time of Plato onwards that we rarely pause even to think about it.

Similarly, Hélèn Cixous sees logos:pathos (masculine/rational:feminine/ emotional) as the most fundamental binary pair, and refers to the privileging of the former over the latter as 'phallocentrism'[9]. Elsewhere, Derrida com-bines the two terms into 'phallogocentrism', which he defines as 'the compli-city of Western metaphysics with a notion of male firstness'[10].

It is no accident that the Greek word 'logos' refers not only to reason (and particularly to the reason of law) but also to the spoken word, since much of Derrida's early work is concerned with what he sees as the unfair privileging of speech over writing (what he sometimes refers to as 'phonocentrism'). In the Christian tradition, the conflation of these two meanings of logos can be traced back to *Genesis*, where God is presented both as the creator of reason out of chaos through the spoken word: 'And God said, Let there be light'[11]; and also *as the spoken word itself*: 'In the beginning was the Word, and the Word was with God, and the Word was God'[12]. In *Of Grammatology*, Derrida pursues this phono/logo/phallocentrism from Plato through to Rousseau and Lévi-Strauss, and returns to it again and again in his later work, for example in *The Post Card* and *Plato's Pharmacy*, where he traces its origins beyond Plato to the ancient Egyptian myth of Theuth. I have already touched upon Derrida's deconstruction of Rousseau, and I shall later explore his deconstruction of the myth of Theuth. For now, however, I shall look briefly at his reading of Lévi-Strauss.

In his book *Tristes Tropiques*, Lévi-Strauss recounts how, by introducing the concept of writing to a 'primitive' tribe of native Americans, he believed that he had propagated their fall from innocence towards the evils of 'modern' society. For Lévi-Strauss, writing initiates and bolsters unequal access to knowledge, and therefore inequality of power; it further leads to the exercise of power from a distance rather than face-to-face democratic debate, thereby corrupting and ultimately destroying the utopian 'primitive' person-to-person culture. Lévi-Strauss was therefore reaffirming the binary pair 'speech:writing' in which writing represents all that is bad and corrupt in society and speech represents all that is innocent and unspoilt.

Derrida's deconstruction of this binary pair consists in exposing the hidden contradictions already prsent in Levi-Strauss' text to demonstrate firstly that the tribe already had a *concept* of writing before Lévi-Strauss arrived (indeed, they even had a word for 'writing'); secondly, that the evils that Lévi-Strauss believed he had brought upon the tribe by the introduction of writing were already there; and thirdly, that the concept of writing (in its broadest sense) cannot, in any case, be separated from the concept of speech. We can see, then, that Derrida's project is not simply to *reverse* the polarity in order to privilege writing over speech. Rather, he wants to show how the two terms are intricately bound together as inseparable parts of a single concept. But he wishes to do more than this; he wants to show how this bifurcation of language into binary pairs influences the way we see the world and, thus, how it shapes the world itself:

> Deconstruction ... analyses and compares conceptual pairs which are currently accepted as self-evident and natural, as if they had not been institutionalised at some precise moment, as if they had no history. Because of being taken for granted they restrict thinking.[13]

We can see, then, that part of the project of deconstruction is to free thinking from the straightjacket of binary pairs by tracing their history and challenging their status as self-evident and natural constructs. The first and most fundamental strategy is therefore to identify logocentrism at work; instances where writers have conceptualised the world in terms of pairs of opposites; and to show how this logocentrism has restricted and distorted thinking and has led to contested conclusions.

We can see this strategy at work in my deconstruction of Raymond Tallis in *Preface 3*. Tallis attempted to set up a binary opposition between evidence-based and evidence-free generalisations. He argued that evidence-based (that is, research-based) generalisations are widely accepted as being the most effective in medicine, therefore they must also be the most effective in all other disciplines, including the arts and humanities; Derrida and the other post-structuralists are therefore not to be trusted because they provide no evidence for their general statements about the world. This 'self-evident and natural' proposition was, you might recall, easily deconstructed by showing how there is no clear-cut dichotomy between evidence-based and evidence-free generalisations, and in particular by demonstrating how Tallis's generalisation from medicine to all other disciplines was itself an evidence-free (and therefore invalid) generalisation. Nevertheless, this 'two cultures' dichotomy continues to dominate and distort thinking in both the arts and the sciences; indeed, it continues to promulgate the very idea that the arts and sciences are in a dynamic tension in which each is struggling for supremacy over the other.

Similarly, in *Deconstruction 1* I try to show how the Evidence-Based Medicine Working Group located its 'new-paradigm:old-paradigm' dichotomy in the well-established phallogocentric opposition between rational: irrational, progressive:backward, scientific:mystical, masculine:feminine, reason:superstition and so on. Thus, simply by attaching to evidence-based medicine (EBM) the label 'new paradigm' (that is, by identifying it as progressive), it is automatically positioned on one side of the divide, thereby attracting all the other positive epithets of phallogocentrism such as scientific, rational, effective, logical and so on. This technique also works in reverse. Consider, for example, the following statement: 'Evidence-based medicine *de-emphasises intuition, unsystematic clinical experience and pathophysiologic rationale* as sufficient grounds for clinical decision making and stresses the examination of evidence from clinical research'[14]. By associating evidence-based practice with all the positive terms of the binary pairs (or, in this case, by distancing it from all the negative terms), it becomes part of the logos, part of the established 'right' way of doing things. EBM is claimed to stand for evidence and research, and against intuition and unsystematic experience. By association, it therefore also stands for logos and hard, scientific, reliable, masculine reason and against pathos and soft, emotional, fallible, feminine intuition. Part of my strategy in deconstructing the paper was therefore to reveal this technique of logocentrism, to question the way in which EBM was sold to the readership of the journal as something new and progressive, and to show how, ultimately, EBM could be rejected as not meeting the very 'evidence-based' criteria that it sought to promote.

In *Deconstruction 2* I show how advocates of evidence-based practice have situated other binary pairs within the framework of logocentrism, most notably quantitative:qualitative research and evidence:experience. But I also offer a way out of logocentrism in Derrida's strategy of *différance* and Lyotard's related concept of the *différend*.

Let's begin with Lyotard:

> As distinguished from a litigation, a differend *[différend]* would be a case of conflict, between (at least) two parties, that cannot be equitably resolved for lack of a rule of judgement applicable to both arguments. One side's legitimacy does not imply the other's lack of legitimacy. However, applying a single rule of judgement to both in order to settle their differend as though it were merely a litigation would wrong (at least) one of them (and both if neither side admits this rule)[15].

A litigation is a case of conflict that can be settled by recourse to some commonly agreed set or rules or criteria. A dispute between two quantitative researchers over the correct size of a sample of respondents would be a litigation that could be resolved by performing a power calculation. Similarly, a dispute between two qualitative researchers over whether data saturation has occurred is a litigation that could be settled by consulting an authoritative text. In contrast, a *différend* occurs where the two parties in dispute cannot agree on the grounds by which their disagreement could be settled. For example, a dispute between a quantitative researcher and a qualitative researcher over the issue of validity could be settled either by applying the criteria of the former, which would disadvantage the latter, or vice versa. There is no independent criterion by which each could be judged fairly against the other, and 'a wrong results from the fact that the rules of the genre of discourse by which one judges are not those of the judged genre or genres of discourse'[16]. The problem, then, is that different discourses employ different criteria against which truth claims are judged, and these criteria are largely incommensurate: 'phrases from heterogeneous regimens cannot be translated from one into the other'[17].

We can see, then, how logocentrism has managed to colonise western thought, and indeed, how evidence-based practice has come to dominate healthcare, since once a particular discourse becomes dominant within a discipline, it settles all *différends* by the application of its own criteria. Thus, in a discipline such as nursing (and increasingly in *all* healthcare disciplines), where the randomised controlled trial is the 'gold standard' for research, all disputes between quantitative and qualitative researchers will be resolved by reference to the rules and standards of the former to the clear disadvantage of the latter. A powerful example of this was given in *Deconstruction 2*, where Kevin Gournay and Sue Ritter observed that:

> There is of course a place for qualitative methods, but such research needs to use a rigorous approach and should be linked to quantitative methodologies ... for it to have any meaning.[18]

Gournay and Ritter further asserted that all qualitative research studies should be subjected to the 'scientific rigour' of quantitative criteria such as interobserver reliability testing and test-retest reliability. Given that such tests are not only irrelevant to qualitative researchers, but are also impossible to implement, it is not surprising that Gournay and Ritter can find very few qualitative studies that meet their standards. For Gournay and Ritter, the conclusion is inescapable: qualitative studies are simply an inferior form of research.

It should by now be coming clear that the problem of the *différend* is not a problem of knowledge but a problem of power; that is, of politics. But it is also a problem of philosophy, 'a philosophical politics apart from the politics of "intellectuals" and of politicians'[19]. In fact, it is the very opposite of the politics of intellectuals: whereas the responsibility of the philosopher lies 'in detecting *différends* and in finding the (impossible) idiom for phrasing them', the intellectual 'is someone who helps forget *différends*, by advocating a given genre, whichever one it may be ... for the sake of political hege-mony'[20]. The intellectual chooses a side, usually that of the dominant dis-course, and when asked to intervene in a dispute, she will judge it according to the rules and criteria of one or other of the parties. For example, when asked to intervene in a *différend* over validity between the qualitative and quantitative researchers, she will apply the criteria of interobserver reliability and test-retest reliability 'for the sake of political hegemony' and the status quo; for the sake of her job and her research funding. The philosopher, on the other hand, will simply point out the presence of the *différend* and the impossibility of judging fairly between the two sides:

> Given 1) the impossibility of avoiding conflicts (the impossibility of indifference) and 2) the absence of a universal genre of discourse to regulate them (or, if you prefer, the inevitable partiality of the judge): to find, if not what can legitimate judgement ... then at least how to save the honour of thinking.[21]

To save the honour of thinking. It is not enough to intellectualise; 'the time has come to philosophise'[22].

It would seem, then, that to philosophise is simply to expose the *différend*; to point out that a fair and considered judgement is not possible; to point out that *any* judgement will, of necessity, favour one side in the dispute over the other. This is perhaps what Derrida intends when he writes of *différance*. Perhaps.

We saw from *Deconstruction 2* that Derrida's solution to the problem of the impossibility of the judgement, of the *différend*, is *différance* (with an a). Derrida noted that the French word *différence* (with an e) takes on two meanings: on the one hand it means *to differ from*, and on the other it means *to defer*. These two actions, of highlighting difference whilst at the same time deferring judgement, are exactly what Derrida is seeking as a resolution to the problem of the binary pair. The difficulty, however, lies in the logic of logocentrism, which allows the word to take on only one meaning at a time. Consider, by way of example, the English verb 'to cleave', which can mean *either* to cut in two or (in its older usage) to join together. Now clearly, when we employ the word in a sentence we can use it to mean *either* to cut *or* to join, but not both at the same time, and it is usually possible to determine the meaning from the context in which it is used. The same applies to the french word *différence*, which can mean *either* to differ from *or* to defer, but not both at once. However, Derrida wanted a word that expressed both meanings at the same time, and he was therefore forced to devise a neologism, an invented word: *différance* (with an a). Or rather, a *neographism*, an invented *written* word, a word whose difference from *différence* only becomes apparent in its written form. Or rather, not a word at all, since, as we have seen, a word can only take one meaning at a time. When I cleave a piece of wood I am either splitting it or joining it, but not both at once. Thus, '*différance* is literally neither a word nor a concept'[23]: not a concept but the 'possibility of conceptuality'[24], a *conceptual process*, a *way* of conceptualising; and not a word, if by word we mean 'the calm, present, and self-referential unity of concept and phonic material'[25]. *Différance* stands outside of formal logic, of formal linguistics, it is 'a hole with indeterminable borders.... In every exposition it would be exposed to disappearing as disappearance. It would risk appearing: disappearing'[26].

Différance, then, has at the same time a temporal meaning and a spatial meaning. It is a deferral in time, a continuous and continual delaying tactic, a strategy by which a final decision need never be made. But it is also a differentiation in space, 'to be not identical, to be other, discernible, etc.'[27]. *Différance* recognises difference but makes no attempt at reconciliation; it simply puts any contested terms *sous rature*, under erasure, by simultaneously writing them in and crossing them out.

To put under erasure: 'to write a word, cross it out, and then print both word and deletion. (Since the word is inaccurate, it is crossed out. Since it is necessary, it remains legible)'[28]. I hinted, suggested perhaps, in *Deconstruc-*

tion 2, that to put a concept under erasure amounts to a philosophical quietism, a simple pointing out of an *aporia*, a *différend*, without recourse to judgement. However, neither Lyotard nor Derrida rules out the possibility of judgement; of making choices in the face of the impossibility of (rational) choice. For Lyotard, the judgement is enigmatic, it follows no rules. How could it, since there *are* no rules that do not do an injustice to one side or the other. Judgements are therefore made ironically, that is, on the understanding that they are indefensible, that there is no logical reason why we should make any particular judgement over any other. But whereas the intellectual suppresses the *differend*, the philosopher faces it, faces the impossibility of a rational, logical choice, and chooses anyway 'to save the honor of thinking'.

Derrida cites Bataille in recognition of this same impossibility: 'These judgements should lead to silence yet I write. This is not paradoxical'[29]. Derrida is insistent that although the ultimate intention of deconstruction is to move *beyond* binary opposites, we should not be too hasty in this operation, since we are dealing here with a 'violent hierarchy' which first needs to be overturned:

> To overlook this phase of overturning is to forget the conflictual and subordinating structure of opposition. Therefore one might proceed too quickly to a *neutralization* that *in practice* would leave the previous opposition, thereby preventing any means of *intervening* in the field effectively.[30]

In *Deconstruction 2*, F criticises R for dwelling too long on simply overturning evidence-based medicine rather than moving on to the next stage of deconstructing the binary pair itself. However, Derrida points out that the simple overturning of the dominant term of the binary pair in favour of the suppressed term is 'an interminable analysis', an analysis that can never end, since 'the hierarchy of dual opposition always reestablishes itself'[31]. The danger, then, when deconstructing a particularly powerful construct such as evidence-based medicine is that, in our desire to see fair play, to represent both sides of the argument, we might simply leave everything as we found it.

Thus, in *Deconstruction 3,* I overturn the binary pair positivism:constructionism by making the latter the dominant term. The next step would be, of course, to move beyond 'the hierarchy of dual opposition'. However, this step is never taken, since positivism/realism exerts such a powerful influence over our thinking that, were I to relax my grip around its throat even for a second, it would surely spring up and reassert its dominance.

And even if or when we finally move beyond a simple overturning of the hierarchy of the binary pair, *différance* is (or perhaps, with Derrida, we should say *différance* is) more than simply the indefinite suspension of meaning; rather 'the thought of *différance* implies the entire critique of classical ontology....'[32]. *Différance* calls into question the very idea of being (or Being) as presence. The fact that we can even *conceive* of *différance* entails a subversion of the classical Aristotelian logic of 'either-or' in favour of a 'neither-either-or-both'. *Différance* therefore challenges *all* dominant discourses by suggesting that there is nothing for them to dominate over; that there is no *dominated*:

> First consequence: *différance* is not. It is not a present being, however excellent, unique, principal, or transcendent. It governs nothing, reigns over nothing, and nowhere exercises any authority. It is not announced by any capital letter. Not only is there no kingdom of *différance*, but *différance* instigates the subversion of every kingdom. Which makes it obviously threatening and infallibly dreaded by everything within us that desires a kingdom, the past or future presence of a kingdom.[33]

This is clearly not a philosophy of quietism, but a challenge, a threat to the logic of being, to what I referred to at the outset of this book as the authority of the 'is', that is, the 'is'. In challenging binary opposites, deconstruction and *différance* threaten statements such as 'validity is...' or 'the gold standard of research is...' by offering the possibility of the privileged term existing *alongside* its opposite. As we have seen, this does not mean that the privileged term is *replaced* by its opposite. Deconstruction does not substitute 'the gold standard of research is the RCT' with 'the gold standard of research is the ethnography'. No, deconstruction questions the entire ontology of being, of presence: 'It is the domination of beings that *différance* everywhere comes to solicit, in the sense that *sollicitare*, in old Latin, means to shake as a whole, to make tremble in entirety'[34].

In keeping with the politico-philosophical nature of deconstruction, Bass refers to this solicitation as 'philosophical-political violence'[35]: 'Every totality ... can be *totally shaken*, that is, can be shown to be founded on that which it excludes, that which would be in *excess* for a reductive analysis of any kind'[36]. And it is in this excess, this residue after the *either* and the *or* have been shaken out, that the ultimate subversive quality of deconstruction lies. As Bass observes, it is 'an excess which cannot be construed within the rules of logic, for the excess can only be conceived a *neither* this *nor* that, or both at the same time - a departure from all rules of logic'[37]. In challenging the 'either-or' logic that underpins all binary pairs, deconstruction shakes the foundation not only of the dominant term of the pair, but of the very concept, the very possibility, of regarding the world in such a way.

Double coding

We have seen how texts can exploit the logocentric logic of binary opposites by privileging one side of the pair at the expense of the other. Whilst this
is a powerful way of asserting authority, sometimes the dominant discourse
finds it necessary to *hide* difference rather than to *exploit* it. One of the ways
that it achieves this is through 'double coding', which is a deliberate strategy
for disguising opposition and dissent within a text. Double coding was first
described by the postmodern architect Charles Jencks as a way of reconcil-
ing the elitist nature of much modern architecture with the demands of the
general public for designs that were more accessible and familiar, that is,
more conservative. Jencks describes how postmodern architects responded
to this challenge by designing buildings that were *at the same time* populist
and elitist, conservative *and* radical. Thus, the untrained eye would see (for
example) a shopping mall designed along (neo)classical lines, whereas the
trained eye would look at the building ironically and pick out subtle archi-
tectural 'codes' designed to subvert the surface classicism. A double coded
building therefore projects 'a mixed message of acceptance and critique'[38].
As Jencks continues, a post-modern[39] architecture is one that '[is] based on
new techniques and old patterns. To simplify, double coding means elite/
popular, accommodating/subversive and new/old'[40]. Thus, as well as asserting authority by dividing the world into binary opposites, power can also be
wielded by blurring and distorting those very same binary pairs. In a market
economy where 'architects must work for the power structure, society at
large, and a client that may have regressive values, tastes or building
motives'[41], they are nevertheless able to subvert this power by 'coding' the
building in a way that can only be read by the trained eye:

> Therefore double coding ... has been adopted as a strategy for
> communicating on various levels at once. Virtually every post-modern
> architect - Robert Venturi, Hans Hollein, Charles Moore, Aldo Rossi, Frank
> Gehry, Arata Isozaki are the notable examples - use popular and elitist
> signs in their work to achieve quite opposite ends.[42]

Jencks continues by noting how other art-forms such as literature and
painting also employ double coding. Thus 'postmodern fiction inscribes itself
within conventional discourses in order to subvert them. It incorporates
cultural realities in order to challenge them: a double coding as strategy'[43].
So, for example, novels such as Umberto Eco's *The Name of the Rose* 'cut
across literary genres and combined such separated types as the historical
romance, comedy, detective story, and philosophical treatise'[44].

Derrida has observed that the same strategy of double coding is
employed in philosophy and other academic disciplines, where it operates
at the level of the single word rather than at the level of form or genre.

Indeed, Derrida himself employs such a strategy by exploiting the multiple meanings of certain words (Spivak calls them 'double-edged words'[45]) in order to demonstrate the 'slipperiness' of the text; to show how there is no fixed relationship between words and what they signify. Similarly, in *Deconstruction 3*, I exploit the multiple meanings of the word 'discourse' and eventually turn it back on itself. Indeed, the entire chapter is a discourse about discourse.

However, whereas Derrida uses such a strategy transparently in order to open up the multiple and often contradictory meanings hidden in all texts, he observes that this double coding can be employed in the service of the dominant discourse in order to obscure these multiple meanings in favour of a single reading that confirms its power and dominance. Just as the post-modern shopping mall is designed to appease the regressive taste and values of the general public whilst at the same time sending a 'secret' message to the *cognoscenti*, so philosophers and other academics deploy certain words duplicitously in order to manipulate the multiple meanings of a text to their own singular and convergent ends.

Derrida refers to such words as 'switches' or 'levers' (recall Spivak's description of 'the positive lever of the signifier'[46]). As he (rather poetically) puts it, 'and I write to you that I love the delicate levers which pass between the legs of a word, between a word and itself to the point of making entire civilizations seesaw'[47]. Or, 'by means of a switch point I will send them elsewhere ... with a stroke of the pen ... I will make everything derail....'[48]. Elsewhere, he refers to such words as *brisures*, or 'hinges', since they function to turn the text in a new direction. Thus, 'The hinge *[brisure]* marks the impossibility that a sign, the unity of a signifier and a signified, be produced within the plenitude of a present and an absolute presence'[49]. But, as we might expect, the word *brisure* is itself a *brisure*, a hinge word that undermines 'the unity of a signifier and a signified', signifying at the same time a hinge or folding joint *and* a fracture or split. The *brisure* unfolds the multiple meanings of the word whilst simultaneously splitting those meanings apart from each other.

The aim of deconstruction is therefore to expose the cynical manipulation and 'closing down' of the text by demonstrating how the multiple meanings of certain words are being suppressed or split off in order to steer the text in a certain direction that favours the ends of the dominant discourse. As Spivak observes:

> If in the process of deciphering a text in the traditional way we come across a word that seems to harbor an unresolvable contradiction, and by virtue of being *one* word is made sometimes to work in one way and sometimes in another and thus is made to point away from the absence

of a unified meaning, we shall catch at that word.... We shall follow its adventures through the text and see the text coming undone as a structure of concealment, revealing its self-transgression, its undecidability.[50]

We have already seen this strategy at work in the introduction to *Deconstruction 2*, where I explored Derrida's deconstruction of Rousseau. In particular, he showed how Rousseau switched between different meanings of the word 'supplement' in order to support his contention that speech is superior to writing; that is, how writing is *supplementary* to speech. But as Derrida demonstrated, the word 'supplement' is a *brisure*, a lever, that signifies not only an *addition to*, but also a *substitute for*. Thus, the suplementarity of writing goes beyond a simple addition to speech and becomes a necessary component of it. Just as the 'colour supplement' is both an addition to the Sunday papers and an integral part of them, in the sense that the concept of the Sunday papers is incomplete without the colour supplement, so writing is both an addition to speech and also an essential part of it.

Derrida's most notable example of how multiple meanings of words can be manipulated and suppressed occurs in the long essay 'Plato's Pharmacy'[51], where he deconstructs Plato's *Phaedrus*, and in particular, Plato's deployment of the word *pharmakon*. A text, then. Or three texts. Perhaps we should say pre-text, con-text and sub-text.

Pre-text: a fragment from the *Phaedrus* in which Plato recounts a conversation between Socrates and the sophist Phaedrus. Phaedrus has enticed Socrates out of the city with the promise of a written text. *Socrates*: 'You must forgive me, dear friend; I'm a lover of learning, and trees and open country won't teach me anything, whereas men in the town do. Yet you seem to have discovered a drug *[pharmakon]* for getting me out'[52].

Writing as a *pharmakon*, a drug to lead Socrates, *he who does not write*, astray. A spoken speech will not do: 'only words that are deferred, reserved, enveloped, rolled up, words that force one to wait for them in the form and under cover of a solid object, letting themselves be desired for the space of a walk, only hidden letters can thus get Socrates moving'[53].

Con-text: Socrates attempts to defend speech against writing by recounting the Egyptian myth of Theuth and Thales. Theuth, the inventor, is a demigod presenting to Thales, king of the gods, his latest invention of writing. 'Here, O King, says Theuth, is a discipline that will make the Egyptians wiser and will improve their memories: both memory and instruction have found their remedy *[pharmakon]*'[54]. Thales, king of the gods, replies:

Theuth, my master of arts, to one man it is given to create the elements of an art, to another to judge the extent of harm and usefulness it will have for those who are going to employ it. And now, since you are father of written letters, your paternal goodwill has led you to pronounce the very opposite of what is their real power. The fact is that this invention will produce forgetfulness in the souls of those who have learned it because they will not need to exercise their memories, being able to rely on what is written, using the stimulus of external marks that are alien to themselves rather than, from within, their own unaided powers to call things to mind. So its not a remedy *[pharmakon]* for memory, but for reminding, that you have discovered. And as for wisdom, you're equipping your pupils only with a semblance of it, not with truth. Thanks to you and your invention, your pupils will be widely read without benefit of a teacher's instruction; in consequence, they'll entertain the delusion that they have wide knowledge, while they are, in fact, for the most part incapable of real judgement. They will also be difficult to get on with since they will be men filled with the conceit of wisdom, not men of wisdom.[55]

So, the king turns the benefits of writing on their head. He is not denying that writing is a *pharmakon*, a drug or potion, but it is a potion that induces evil: it is a *poison* rather than a *remedy*.

Sub-text: The axis of the paper, around which all three texts revolve, is the *pharmakon*. As Derrida points out, the word is polysemic, it has a number of meanings, several of which are incommensurate, indeed, contradictory. It is at once a potion, a drug, a remedy and a poison, and whenever we encounter the word, we should therefore bear all these meanings in mind: not *pharmakon*, but *pharmakon*. The difficulty, though, comes when we attempt to translate the word from Greek into (say) French or English. However we translate it, we necessarily loose its polysemic meaning: if we render it as 'remedy', then we lose the meaning of 'poison' and *vice versa*. But the problem runs far deeper: Derrida observes that Plato was himself involved in a translation 'between Greek and Greek; a violent difficulty in the transference of a nonphilosopheme into a philosopheme. With this problem of translation we will thus be dealing with nothing less than the problem of the very passage into philosophy'[56].

For Derrida, then, Plato's handling of the word *pharmakon* is a deliberate attempt to subvert its multiple meanings, an attempt to subject the word to the dialectical Aristotelian rigour of either/or, to reduce it to a single meaning, that is, to translate it into the language of philosophy, into a *philosopheme*. And for Plato, whose project is to elevate speech above writing, this means cynically and deliberately emphasising the meaning of *pharmakon* as 'poison' above its meaning as 'remedy': writing, then, is a poison. Thus: 'All translations into languages that are the heirs and depositaries of Western metaphysics thus produce on the *pharmakon* an *effect of analysis* that violently destroys it, reduces it to one of its simple elements by interpreting it, paradoxically enough, in the light of the ulterior developments it itself has made possible'[57].

Here, then, is the *brisure*, the hinge, the splitting off, the double coding. Theuth wishes to present writing in a positive light; he therefore presents it as a *pharmakon*, a *remedy* against forgetfulness. Thus:

> He *turns* the word on its strange and invisible pivot, presenting it from a single one, the most reassuring, of its *poles*. This medicine is beneficial; it repairs and produces, accumulates and remedies, increases knowledge and reduces forgetfulness. Its translation by 'remedy' nonetheless erases, in going outside the Greek language, the other pole reserved in the word *pharmakon*.[58]

Theuth turns the meaning of the text on the pivot, the *brisure*, of the word *pharmakon* by deliberately emphasising one aspect of its meaning at the expense of all the others. But Thales plays him at his own game; writing is indeed a *pharmakon*, a drug, but it is a harmful drug, a *poison*. At a stroke, a twist of the hinge, the text is sent in the opposite direction. Similarly, Plato's own description of writing plays on the same double code. 'You seem to have discovered a drug *[pharmakon]* for getting me out', he tells Phaedrus. He *suggests* that writing is a remedy, but we can see from the context of his recounting of the myth of Theuth that he is *implying* that it is, in reality, a poison.

We are dealing here with subtle forces. The translation from Greek into English offers no indication of these multiple meanings. Here we see the word 'remedy', there we see the word 'poison'; there is nothing to suggest that they are, in fact, the same Greek word. But Derrida sees the same forces at work in the translation of words from their everyday usage into philosophical texts, from 'nonphilosophemes' into 'philosophemes'. Thus, philosophers (and academics in general) see polysemy as a threat, as meaning run riot and as something outside of their control. It is therefore something to be tamed, but also to be used. Polysemic words, words that contain several incommensurate meanings, are able to be bent, to be twisted on their hinges first one way and then the other, their double (multiple) codes exploited by the academic to steer the text in whichever direction suits her from moment to moment. And it is the exposure of this subtle but powerful manipulation of polysemic words that comprises Derrida's second strategy for deconstruction.

We saw this double coding at work in *Deconstruction 2*, where the polysemic nature of the word 'evidence' was explored. You will recall, then, how David Thompson, in his paper *Why evidence-based nursing*, began with the standard definition of evidence-based nursing as 'integrating research evidence with clinical expertise, the resources available and the views of patients'[59]. However, from offering a broad and widely accepted definition in the first sentence, he then used the word 'evidence' as a *brisure* to switch the paper to a discussion about barriers to *research*-based practice, and the word 'evidence' was not used again until the final sentence, which switched back once again to conclude that 'significant progress has been made in helping nurses to take an evidence-based approach to decisions about care'. In this way, Thompson was able to discuss the well-documented strategies for overcoming the barriers to *research*-based practice whilst neatly sidestepping the far more problematic barriers to implementing the broader concept of evidence.

Interestingly, in the very same week Mike Nolan and colleagues published a paper entitled 'Evidence-based care: can we overcome the barriers?'[60] which again introduced the term 'evidence-based care' in the first sentence, before going on to discuss barriers to *research*-based practice. In both cases, the term 'evidence' was used to switch the focus of the debate back and forth between research and clinical expertise/available resources/patients' views as and when it suited the writers.

Perhaps these were simple oversights; perhaps these eminent professors of nursing simply did not realise that they had both written papers with 'evidence based practice' in the title that looked exclusively at *research*-based practice. Or perhaps they did. Perhaps the contradictions represent a cynical exercise in double coding, in which two different messages for two different audiences are simultaneously transmitted in the same text. In this case, the overt message to practitioners is that their clinical expertise is still valued by evidence-based practice, whilst the coded message to researchers and academics is that research findings remain by far the most important source of evidence. Practitioners are therefore pacified by a definition of evidence-based practice that includes clinical expertise and patients' views, whilst academics are reassured that the real power for clinical decision making rests with them.

We saw this same double coding at work in the use of the words 'authority' and 'expert'. According to the precepts of evidence-based medicine, authoritarian practice (that is, practice based on experience and expertise) is to be discouraged. Thus, the Evidence-Based Medicine Working Group claimed that EBM 'puts a much lower value on authority'[61], which is replaced by evidence from research, whilst Davidoff et al added that 'practising physicians increasingly expect, and are expected, to base their decisions on "the evidence" rather than on authority'[62]. DiCenso, Cullum and Ciliska, the editors of the journal *Evidence-Based Nursing* also cited some examples of where practice based on the authority of experts has later been shown by research to be flawed, including:

The use of cover gowns by nurses when caring for normal newborns in the nursery, and shaving before surgery. Few of us would want to begin a drug regimen that has not been proved to be safe and effective in an RCT.[63]

Practice based on so-called expert authority is therefore bad, dangerous and overly subjective.

Or is it? In my deconstruction of DiCenso, Cullum and Ciliska's journal *Evidence-Based Nursing*, I attempted to show how the authority of the practitioner has been replaced by the authority of the academic researcher, whose role includes 'to identify ... the best ... articles', 'to summarise this literature in the form of structured abstracts', 'to provide brief, *highly expert* comment' and 'to disseminate the summaries in a timely fashion to nurses'[64]. It would appear, then, that clinical experts cannot be trusted: they are overly subjective, they make mistakes, they misuse their power and authority. However, academic and methodological experts are not, it seems, subject to the same limitations: they can be trusted absolutely, are completely objective in their decision making, never make mistakes, never falsify their findings, and would not dream of misusing their power and authority.

We can see that the words 'authority' and 'expertise' are used to switch the focus of the discourse, and far from *replacing* authority with evidence, the expertise and authority of the clinical practitioner has simply been replaced by the expertise and authority of the academic researcher. As Feinstein and Horwitz observe, 'interpretive decisions by old pre-EBM experts may be replaced by interpretive decisions from a new group of experts with EBM "credentials"'[65]. And although it might be argued that the new experts are basing their judgements on pre-defined criteria rather than personal experience, 'the use of those criteria will involve subtle judgements and decisions from the large panel of experts whose identities and credentials may be difficult to discern'[66]. Far from being *freed* from the tyranny of authority and unvalidated expertise, the strategy of double coding is employed by academics to replace one source of authority with another: their own.

Writing *of*, *in* and *at* the margins

Deconstruction is writing, but as we saw in *Preface 2*, writing for Derrida is concerned not only with content, but also with form and style. Indeed, they are intimately linked such that each determines and is determined by the others. For example, Derrida's book *The Postcard* takes as its subject matter a particular picture postcard of Plato and Socrates (content), it is presented as a series of postcards, each dated and (literally) addressed to a specific recipient (form), and it is written informally as one might write a postcard (style). Thus, 'By publishing that which, concerning the postcard, looks like a "post card"....'[67].

We can see this symbiotic relationship between content, form and style most clearly in Derrida's treatment of the theme of the margin, which has been a constant preoccupation throughout his writing. Starting, then, with content: much of Derrida's work has been concerned with the *subject* of margins, that is, with the borders between disciplines (most notably, the border between philosophy and other genres such as literature and art), and with the borders between text and non-text. For example:

> If we are to approach a text, it must have an edge. The question of the text ... has not merely 'touched' 'shore', *le bord*, all those boundaries that form the running border of what used to be called a text, of what we once thought this word could identify, i.e., the supposed end and beginning of a work, the unity of a corpus, the title, the margins, the signatures, the referential realm outside the frame, and so forth. What has happened, is a sort of overrun *[débordement]* that spoils all these boundaries and divisions and forces us to extend the accredited concept, the dominant notion of a 'text', of what I still call a 'text', for strategic reasons, in part - a 'text' that is henceforth no longer a finished corpus of writing, some content enclosed in a book or its margins, but a differential network, a fabric of traces referring endlessly to something other than itself, to differential traces.[68]

That is not to say that the text has no borders, that all the world is nothing but text (a common misreading of Derrida), but rather '...to work out the theoretical and practical system of these margins, these borders, once more, from the ground up'[69].

Following Derrida, the text you are now reading has also sought to re-inscribe the margins of the book through experimenting with its structure (three prefaces, three afterwords), with its ending and beginning (where does this book end; where does it begin?), with the referential realm (deconstruction as an address to an imaginary Audience, as a series of letters to an imaginary Reader, as a discourse about discourse in the form of a discourse) and through attempting to blur its authorship, its signature (who wrote what; does it matter?).

But as well as taking the margin as its *subject*, Derrida's writing is also concerned with *marginalia*, with footnotes and asides or with tiny and seemingly inconsequential fragments of text (Spivak's 'promising marginal text'[70]). Sometimes this involves picking up on insignificant snippets: a passage from Nietzsche[71]; a passing remark from Heidegger 'in the margins of *Sein und Zeit*'[72]; a brief note by Foucault on a brief note by Descartes. Thus:

My point of departure might appear slight and artificial. In this 673-page book, Michel Foucault devotes three pages - and, moreover, in a kind of prologue to his second chapter - to a certain passage from the first of Descartes's *Meditations*.... [T]he sense of Foucault's entire project can be pinpointed in these few allusive and somewhat enigmatic pages...[73]

Elsewhere, Derrida muses on a medieval engraving which appears to have transposed the names of Plato and Socrates[74]; on an obscure point in an obscure correspondence between Heidegger and the art critic Schapiro about whether a pair of shoes in a painting by Van Gogh really was a *pair*[75]; on a six-line poem by Francis Ponge[76]; on the three-word sentence *'Il aura obligé'* by Levinas[77]; on the single word 'yes' in Joyce's *Ulysses*; and ultimately, on nothing, on what is *missing* from Heidegger's *Sein und Zeit*.

And we can see a similar focus on marginalia in this book, where I deconstruct (amongst other things) an application for membership to a professional body; the (impossible) act of deconstruction itself; a(nother) poem by Francis Ponge; the title and authorship (authority) of a paper; the aims of a journal; a fragment of conversation between a therapist and his client; the sentence 'A new paradigm for medical practice is emerging'; the word 'community'; and ultimately, like Derrida, nothing, the absence of a question mark (and the absence of a colon in the deconstruction of the absence of a question mark).

As well as focussing on marginalia, *Deconstruction 3* also addresses issues that are considered to be on the margins of the discourse of healthcare (indeed, on the margins of what it is permissible to *think* in the discourse of healthcare), such as masturbation and sexual relationships between patient and client. But as we have seen, the aim of deconstruction (if it can be said to have an aim) is not to replace the 'no sex' dictum with its opposite. I am not arguing *for* sexual promiscuity between therapist and client, but rather calling the dictum itself into question. I am not challenging accepted views, but challenging the very discourse that invests power in so-called accepted views; indeed, that authorises their acceptance.

But as we have seen, in deconstructive writing, content and form often reflect one another. To paraphrase Derrida, then, that which concerns the margin should also look like the margin, just as in Deconstruction 3, that which concerns discourse also looks like a discourse. Thus, we have seen that much of Derrida's writing is *literally* in the margins insofar as it is physically placed on the edge of the page. So, for example, his book *Margins of Philosophy* begins with the essay 'Tympan', in which two texts are presented side by side as columns of text, along with elaborate footnotes running across the bottom of the page. As Kamuf points out (you will recall from *Preface 2*):

By means of these typographics, Derrida contrives to proliferate the margins on which and in which he is writing. In its much narrower column, the Leiris quotation appears to be written in the margin of Derrida's column on the left, whereas the space between the two is a thin blank column running down the right third of the page.[78]

You have perhaps noticed several similar attempts to write 'in the margins' in this book. For example, *Deconstruction 1* presents a key text on evidence-based medicine on the left side of the page, with my deconstruction of it as a sort of right-hand margin. Similarly in *Deconstruction 2*, a text on the left that is a deconstruction of evidence-based nursing is itself deconstructed in the right-hand margin.

But as well as writing *of* and *in* the margins, Derrida also writes *at* the margins ('I try to keep myself at the *limit* of philosophical discourse'[79]), at the border between philosophy and literature. And as before, content and form merge. Thus, in a margin beneath the main text, Derrida writes:

> I wish to pose the question of the *bord*, the edge, the border, and the *bord de mer*, the shore.... The question of the borderline precedes, as it were, the determination of all the dividing lines that I have just mention-ed: between a fantasy and a 'reality', an event and a nonevent, a fiction and a reality, one corpus and another, and so forth.[80]

An interrogation of the border between fact and fiction, truth and fantasy. Elsewhere, then, the question: 'What is literature? And first of all, what is writing? How does writing come to upset even the question 'What is?' and even 'What does that mean?'[81]. The question 'what is?'; the question of identity and of truth. So how does literature (and Derrida) come to upset this question?

Whereas the traditional aim of philosophy is the search for a universal truth (that is, a metaphysics), a search which Derrida considers to be fruitless, literature is concerned with the particular, the singular. Thus: 'something literary will have begun when it will not have been possible to decide if, when I speak of something I speak of some thing, of the thing itself....'[82]. A philosophical enquiry might be concerned with ontology, the nature of Being. However, a literary enquiry would concern itself with narrative, the nature of a *particular* being. For a philosopher to write at the border between literature and philosophy is thus to question, to undermine, the *very function* of philosophy, the quest for universal truth. Derrida's project, then, is to deconstruct philosophy from the inside by writing in such a way that subverts its claim for universality; that is, by writing 'unphilosophically'. As Kamuf observes:

Derrida's *concern* with literature is not that of the philosopher. This means, to begin with, that he does not ask the philosopher's question: 'What is (literature)?' which subjects the literary, the poetic to a concept. His concern, rather, is precisely with how the philosopher's question is dislocated, thrown off balance by a writing practice that does not claim to represent some truth outside itself and thus does not attempt to hide its own inscription. It is, then, this practice that is allowed to interrogate - indirectly, discretely - the very distinctions supposed by philosophy to divide one kind of writing from another.[83]

The aim of deconstructive writing is not to discover universal truth but rather to interrogate the very distinction erected by philosophy between writing that is and is not philosophical. If deconstruction is concerned with speaking not of something, but rather of some *thing*, not with what is, but with what is, with representation, then deconstructive writing is freed from asserting the authority of the 'is'. Some of the consequences of that freedom are explored in the second Afterword.

Notes

1 Derrida, J. The Time of a Thesis: Punctuations. In A. Montefiore (ed) *Philosophy in France Today*, Cambridge: Cambridge University Press, 1983, pp.40-1

2 Woltreys, J. *Deconstruction.Derrida*, Basingstoke: Macmillan, 1998

3 Derrida, J. 'As if I were Dead': An Interview with Jacques Derrida. In J. Brannigan, R. Robbins and J. Wolfreys (eds) *Applying: to Derrida*, London: Macmillan, 1996, p.218

4 Derrida, J. (1987) Letter to a Japanese Friend. In P. Kamuf (ed) *A Derrida Reader: Reading Between the Blinds*, New York: Harvester Wheatsheaf, 1991, p.273

5 Derrida, J. The Time is Out of Joint. In A. Haverkamp (ed) *Deconstruction is/in America: A New Sense of the Political*, New York: New York University Press, 1995, p.15

6 McQuillan, M. Introduction: Five Strategies for Deconstruction. In M. McQuillan (ed) *Deconstruction: A Reader*, Edinburgh: Edinburgh University Press, 2000, p.5

7 Derrida, J. 'The Time of a Thesis: Punctuations, op. cit., p.40

8 Spivak, G.C. Translator's Preface. In J. Derrida *Of Grammatology*, Baltimore: The Johns Hopkins University Press, 1974, p.lxxvii

9 Cixous, H. Sorties: Out and Out: Attacks/Ways Out/Forays. In H. Cixous and C. Clement *The Newly Born Woman*, Minneapolis: University of Minnesota Press, 1986

10   Derrida, J. (1982) Choreographies. In P. Kamuf, op. cit., p.445

11   Holy Bible, *Genesis* 1:3, King James Version

12   Holy Bible, *John* 1:1, King James Version

13   Derrida, J. Architetture ove il desiderio può abitare, *Domus*, 671, April
     1986. Cited by Benjamin in M. McQuillan, op. cit., p.223

14   Evidence-Based Medicine Working Group. Evidence-based medicine: a
     new approach to teaching the practice of medicine, *JAMA*, 1992, 268,
     17, 2420-5, my emphasis

15   Lyotard, J.-F. (1983) *The Differend: Phrases in Dispute*, Minneapolis:
     University of Minnesota Press, 1988, p.xi

16   Ibid., p.xi

17   Ibid., p.xii

18   Gournay, K. & Ritter, S. What future for research in mental health nursing:
     a rejoinder to Parsond, Beech and Rolfe, *Journal of Psychiatric and
     Mental Health Nursing*, 1998, 5, 227-230, p.228

19   Lyotard, op. cit., p.xiii

20   Ibid., p.142

21   Ibid., p.xii

22   Ibid., p.xiii

23   Derrida, J. (1968) Différance. In *Margins of Philosophy*, New York:
     Harvester, 1982, p.3

24   Ibid., p.11

25   Ibid., p.11

26   Ibid., p.6

27   Ibid., p.8

28   Spivak, op. cit., p.xiv

29   Cited in J. Derrida, *Writing and Difference*, Chicago: University of
     Chicago Press, 1978, p.262

30   Derrida, J. (1972) *Positions*, London: Athlone Press, 1982, p.42

31   Ibid., p.42

32   Derrida, J. (1968) Différance, op. cit., p.21

33   Ibid., pp.21-2

34   Ibid., p.21

35   Bass, A. Translator's Introduction. In J. Derrida *Writing and Difference*,
     London: Routledge & Kegan Paul, 1978, p.xvi

36   Ibid., p.xvi

37   Ibid., pp.xvi-xvii

38   Jencks, C. *What is Post-Modernism?*, Chichester: John Wiley & Sons,
     1996, p.30

39 Notice that the discipline of architecture usually inserts a hyphen between the 'post' and the 'modern'

40 Ibid., p.30

41 Ibid., p.30

42 Ibid., p.34

43 Ibid., p.32

44 Ibid., p.32

45 Spivak, op. cit., p.xlix

46 Ibid., p.lxxvii

47 Derrida, J. (1980) *The Post Card*, Chicago: University of Chicago Press, 1987, p.78

48 Ibid., p.177

49 Derrida, J. (1967) *Of Grammatology*, Baltimore: The Johns Hopkins University Press, 1974, p.69

50 Spivak, op. cit., p.lxxv

51 Derrida, J. (1972) *Dissemination*, London: The Athlone Press, 1981

52 Ibid., p.71

53 Ibid., p.71

54 Ibid., pp.96-7

55 Ibid., p.102

56 Ibid., p.72

57 Ibid., p.99, his emphasis

58 Ibid., p.97, his emphasis

59 Thompson, D. Why evidence-based nursing, *Nursing Standard*, 1998, 13, 9, 58-9

60 Nolan, M., Morgan, L., Curran, M., Clayton, J., Gerrish, K. & Parker, K. Evidence-based care: can we overcome the barriers?, *British Journal of Nursing*, 1998, 7, 20, 1273-8

61 Evidence-Based Medicine Working Group. Evidence-based medicine: a new approach to teaching the practice of medicine, *JAMA*, 1992, 268, 17, 2420-5

62 Davidoff, F., Case, K. & Fried, P.W. Evidence-based medicine: why all the fuss?, *Annals of Internal Medicine*, 1995, 122, 9, 727

63 DiCenso, A., Cullum, N. & Ciliska, D. Implementing evidence-based nursing: some misconceptions, *Evidence-Based Nursing*, 1998, 1, 2, 38-430

64 These aims of the journal can be found on page 2 of any edition

65 Feinstein, A.R. & Horwitz, R.I. Problems in the "evidence" of evidence-based medicine, *The American Journal of Medicine*, 1997, 103, 529-35

66   Ibid., p.534
67   Derrida, J. (1980) *The Post Card*, Chicago: University of Chicago Press, 1987
68   Derrida, J. Living On: Border Lines. In H. Bloom et al, *Deconstruction and Criticism*, London: Routledge & Kegan Paul, 1979, pp.83-4
69   Ibid., p.84
70   Spivak, op. cit., p.lxxvii
71   Derrida (1978) Spurs: Nietzsche's Styles. In Kamuf, op. cit., p.353
72   Derrida (1987) Geschlecht: Sexual Difference, Ontological Difference. In Kamuf, op. cit. p.383
73   Derrida (1964) Cogito and the History of Madness. In J. Derrida, *Writing and Difference*, op. cit., p.32, my italics
74   Derrida, *The Postcard*, op. cit.
75   Derrida (1978) The Truth in Painting. In Kamuf, op. cit.
76   Derrida (1987) Psyche: Inventions of the Other. In Kamuf, ibid., p.201
77   Derrida (1987) At This Very Moment in This Work Here I Am. In Kamuf, ibid., p.405
78   Kamuf, ibid., p.146
79   Derrida, J. (1972) *Positions*, London: The Athlone Press, 1987, p.6
80   Derrida, (1979) Living On: Border Lines, op. cit., pp. 82-3
81   Derrida, J. Ponctuations: le temps de la thèse, *Du Droit à la Philosophie*, Paris: Galilée, 1990, p.443
82   Derrida, J. *Passions*, Paris: Galilée, 1993, p.89
83   Kamuf, op. cit., pp.143-4

Afterword 2

Writing in the margins

It is because writing is inaugural, in the fresh sense of the word, that it is dangerous and anguishing. It does not know where it is going, no knowledge can keep it from the essential precipitation towards the meaning that it constitutes and that is, primarily, its future.[1]

Just begin, then...
Deconstruction is writing, but a specific kind of writing; the aim of deconstructive writing is not the pursuit of universal truth, but to discover, to uncover, the particular truth inside myself. Writing myself, then. Responding not so much to the text as to what the text is invoking in me, deep in my self. 'The writer's thought does not control his language from without; the writer is himself a kind of new idiom, constructing itself'[2]. Or: I am writing a text and I call it GR. A text, as Derrida tells us, that does not know where it is going, but that nothing can keep from its destination. Hélène Cixous observes: 'At times I prepare myself to say; "I have some things to say" I say to myself. This is how I prepare my seminar during two or three days. When the day comes it does not at all happen as planned: what I say is infinitely far from what I had counted on saying'[3]. Or, as Edmond Jabès adds, 'The art of the writer consists in little by little making words interest themselves in his books'[4].

I must trust in writing, then, trust that words will become interested in my book, I must simply start and pray for the best: 'This page writes itself without help, it is

Some notes on writing Writing is at the interface between theory and practice. It is a one-way street between theoreticians and practitioners. For most practitioners, it is the only link to researchers (although, as I said, it is predominantly a one-way link). Writing is the lifeblood of any academic discipline. It is impossible to imagine a discipline without writing.

Writing is also the imposition of power. Writing is therefore seen as dangerous in the wrong hands. Writing is monitored and controlled by a select and (largely) self-elected group which imposes form, style and content on writing. The closer the monitoring (in the form of so-called 'peer review'), the higher the status given to the writing. The reason that books are awarded less academic status than peer reviewed journal papers is because the power elite has less control over the production and dissemination of books. Books are monitored and controlled by the market. The power of books is devalued and undermined by criticising them as not being peer-reviewed (and therefore as containing uncertain knowledge).

proof of the existence of gods'[5]. The first sentence of the book, of the chapter, of the page, is a prayer to the god of writing.

The first sentence, then. Not the first word, not the first paragraph, *the first sentence*.

> Enter a sentence. And there was the book. And it had never before been seen.
> From sentence to sentence we leap.
> I adore the multiple powers of sentences. Often the events of my life come in sentences or are sentences.[6]

Or:

> Valéry said: 'One does not think words, one thinks only sentences'. He said it because he was a writer. A writer is not someone who expresses his thoughts, his passion, or his imagination in sentences, but someone who thinks in sentences: A Sentence-Thinker.[7]

The writer thinks in sentences; she thinks in the form, structure and grammar of the book, of the text. I must think in the language of writing, not in the language of speech:

> But how is it that I do not speak that language of writing when I speak? I cannot write in the air with my voice? When I speak - no writing, only discourse.[8]

The form, the structure and the grammar of the thought *shapes* the content of the thought; the form of expression of the thought shapes the thought itself; the medium is the message. Or, the way I write determines what I say. Clearly. If I write two parallel texts, if I write in three different fonts, if I write in a style that is less than formal, it is not to impress or to confuse; it is because the text demands it. If I think in sentences, then I also think in commas and semi-colons, in Arial and in Times New Roman, in columns and in footnotes.

Spacing, framing, punctuation, type style, layout, and other nonphonetic structures of difference constitute the material interface of writing. Traditional literary and linguistic research overlooks such graphic forms, focusing instead on the Word as the center of communication.[9]

The page is not a neutral background to the text, not simply a space on which to inscribe meaning. The page is *part of* the text; text and page together form a landscape of varying forms and text(ure)s.

A landscape, then. Sky, sea and stones. Gas, liquid and solid. At each transition the atoms become more bound together, more rigid, less free. Writing starts in freedom and ends in discipline. It just starts; only later do we tie it down, solidify it, polish it up.

So, begin in freedom. But where? At the beginning, of course. We might say, at the upper edge.

If we are to approach *[aborder]* a text, for example, it must have a *bord*, an edge. Take this text. What is its upper edge? Its title? But when do you start reading it? What if you started reading it after the first sentence (another upper edge), which functions as its first reading head but which itself in turn folds its outer edges back over onto inner edges whose mobility - multilayered, quotational, displaced from meaning to meaning - prohibits you from making out a shoreline? There is a regular *sub-merging* of the shore.[10]

I must therefore consider not only *what* I intend to write (that is, the content of the text), not only *how* I intend to write it (that is, the style of the text), but also with *where* I intend to write (that is, the form of the text), with where exactly on the page I will place my text, with how I will present it to the reader, with how I will frame the landscape that is my text. The design of the text is something that I cannot ignore. The medium *is* the message: the austere layout of the academic journal tells me that the texts published here are serious, that they mean business; the more reader-friendly layout of the professional journal tells me that these texts are themselves friendly and willing to engage in dialogue with me.

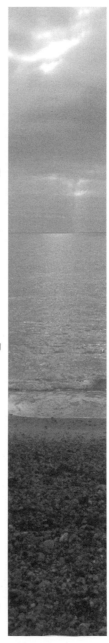

Most researchers and many theoreticians see communication as the most important (indeed, as the only) function of academic writing. For them, writing should be clear and unambiguous. It should convey a single (simple) message. Writing (for them) is largely prescriptive. When it is discursive, the debates are usually resolved (closed) by the writer. This form of writing presumes a simple model of communication in which the message proceeds without complication from the mind of the writer to her pen, and hence to the eyes and mind of the reader.

So how to begin? Just begin, you say, trust in the text; the texture; or, as Roland Barthes put it, the *grain*; the grain of the voice. Barthes says I should *write aloud*, 'which is nothing like speech'[11]:

> ...*writing aloud* is not phonological but phonetic; its aim is not the clarity of messages, the theater of emotions; what it searches for (in a perspective of bliss) are the pulsational incidents, the language lined with flesh, a text where we can hear the grain of the throat, the patina of consonants, the voluptuousness of vowels, a whole carnal stereophony: the articulation of the body, of the tongue, not that of meaning, of language.[12]

Writing with/from my body. It is perhaps no accident that the form of the book mimics the form of the body:
body - the main or central part of printed or written matter;
figure - a diagram or pictorial representation in a text;
head - a word often in larger letters placed above a passage in order to introduce or categorise it;
gloss - a brief explanation, e.g., in the margin of a text, of a difficult word or expression (from the Greek *glossa*, tongue);
spine - the back of a book, usually lettered with the title and author's name;
footnote - a note of reference, explanation, or comment typically placed at the bottom of a printed page;
appendix - a supplement ... attached at the end of a book or other piece of writing[13].
Write the grain of the throat, then, 'the language lined with flesh', the very texture of language, which, Barthes tells us, takes precedence over meaning.

So where, then, does meaning originate, if not with the author of the text(ure)?

> *Text* means *Tissue*; but whereas hitherto we have always taken this tissue as a product, a ready-made veil, behind which lies, more or less hidden, meaning (truth), we are now emphasizing, in the tissue, the generative idea that the text is made, is worked out in a perpetual interweaving; lost in this tissue - this texture - the subject unmakes himself, like a spider dissolving the constructive secretions of its web.[14]

The author is dead, the subject unmade, to be reconstructed by the *reader*. I write, then, to be *read*; that
the reader might also be a writer. Not to be read, but
to be *read*. Not a readerly *(lisible)* text, one that cannot
be rewritten, cannot be interpreted. Rather, a writerly
(scriptible) text, one that stimulates, challenges, con-
fronts: 'a *writerly* text is one that I read with difficulty,
unless I completely transform my reading regime'[15].

A writerly text, then, one to force you to transform
your reading regime; to read in a different way; that is,
to see the world in a different way. And yet, I must
remember that I am not just writing; I am writing a
book, a work, an *oeuvre*, 'a piece of merchandise'[16].
Thus: 'While I write, the writing is thereby at every
moment flattened out, banalized, made guilty by the
work to which it must eventually contribute'[17]. How am I
to write, then?

> Why, *blindly*. At every moment of the effort, lost,
> bewildered, and driven, I can only repeat to myself
> the words which end Sartre's *No exit:* let's go on.[18]

I must write blindly. Which reminds me, of course (how
could it not?), of Hélène Cixous, who was so myopic
that she could *literally* not see beyond the end of her
nose:

> I owe a large part of my writing to my nearsighted-
> ness. I am a woman. But before being a woman I
> am a myope. Myopia is my secret.[19]

I must write blindly:

> Whenever I go off (writing is first of all a departure, an
> embarkation, an expedition) I slip away from the
> diurnal world and diurnal sociality, with a simple
> magic trick: I close my eyes, my ears. And *presto*: the
> moorings are broken. At that instant I am no longer of
> this political world. It is no more. Behind my eyelids I
> am Elsewhere. Elsewhere there reigns the other light. I
> write by the other light. When I close my eyes the
> passage opens, the dark gorge, I descend.[20]

Others write to provoke a response (other than as a prescription to write in a certain way) rather than to communicate a message. For them, writing should be obscure and open. It should avoid proclaiming a single and obvious message. It is concerned with asking rather than answering questions. It engages the reader in a creative partnership (although sometimes covertly). It is catalytic rather than communicative. Writing is therefore dangerous. It incites, it subverts, it deconstructs. Writing is at the interface between theory and practice. The way that a discipline writes itself determines the kind of practice it strives to promote.

We will use this

ladder, travelling

along the steps,

the   moments,

like periods, eras,

airs,   epochs,

leading   toward

the   deepest.

Toward   what   I

call: the   truth,

toward what calls

me, attracts me

magnetically,

i r r e s i s t i b l y

Barthes also descends into his writing: 'The closer I come to the work, the deeper I descend into writing; I approach its unendurable depth...'[21]. For Cixous, writing is a ladder, not the descent itself, but the *means* of her descent, of her exploration of the deep:

> To us, this ladder has a *descending* movement, because we ordinarily believe the descent is easy. The writers I love are *descenders*, explorers of the lowest and deepest. [...] When we climb up toward the bottom, we proceed carried in the direction of - we're searching for something: the unknown. [22]

But searching for what? Cixous continues, 'Toward what I call: *the truth*, toward what calls me, attracts me magnetically, irrestistibly'[23]. Towards myself. 'You do not write what you know, but what you are un-aware you know and then discover, without surprise, you have always known'[24]. A descent into the sub-conscious, then. I write so that I might know *myself*.

But how to begin? Make a pot of tea, sit at your desk, and *write*, you say. With Flaubert, then, 'One can only think and write sitting down'. But of course. Or with Nietzsche:

> Here I have got you, you nihilist! A sedentary life is the real sin against the Holy Spirit. Only those thoughts that come to you when you are walking have any value.[25]

And Cixous:

> Mandelstam asks very seriously in his 'Conversa-tion about Dante' how many pairs of shoes Dante must have worn out in order to write *The Divine Comedy*, because, he tells us, that could only have been written on foot, walking without stopping, which is also how Mandelstam wrote.[26]

Perhaps, then, I should write as I walk (quickly, purposefully, without looking about me).

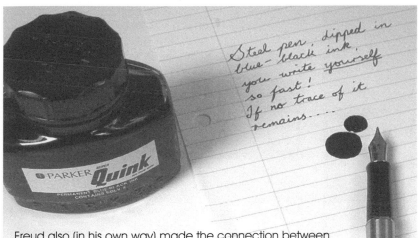

Steel pen, dipped in
blue-black ink,
you write yourself
so fast!
If no trace of it
remains.....

Freud also (in his own way) made the connection between writing and walking:

> As soon as writing, which entails making a liquid flow out of a tube on to a piece of white paper, assumes the significance of copulation, or as soon as walking becomes a symbolic substitute for treading upon the body of mother earth, both writing and walking are stopped because they represent the performance of a forbidden sexual act.[27]

For Freud, then, writing represents a forbidden sexual act. The flow of liquid from a tube. So writing, *forbidden* writing, writing *myself* (think again of Rousseau's dangerous supplement) cannot happen on a computer.

> I am not an intellectual. I am a painter. No computers. You do not paint with a computer. I paint, I draw the sentences from the secret well. I paint the passage: one cannot speak it. One can only perform it. No, never computers.[28]

True, reflective, reflexive, exploratory, descending, deconstructive writing only happens with a pen. Whilst walking. In sentences. At the edge. In the margin. Unexpectedly. Without help. But where to start? With the first sentence; a prayer to (the god of) writing.

'And the "you write yourself so fast" is thus the mark of a reflection...'

Derrida - Points..., p.367

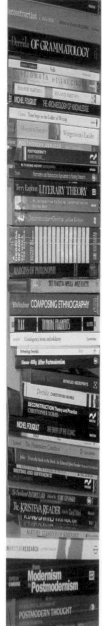

'I'll get on, then.'

'That would be nice,' you say. 'All that you have done so far in this book is to quote other people.'

'"I quote others only the better to express myself",'[29] I reply.

'There, you're doing it again.'

'You're right, I am. Now that I think about it, almost everything I've written has previously been said by someone else. I don't seem to have an original thought in my head.'

'Just as I thought...'

'Perhaps Barthes was right, then, when he wrote "The text is a tissue of quotations drawn from the innumerable centres of culture ... the writer can only imitate a gesture that is always anterior, never original. His only power is to mix writings, to counter the ones with the others, in such a way as never to rest on any of them"[30].'

'Isn't that what they call "Intertext"?'

'Ah, yes, intertext. "The act of reading ... plunges us into a network of textual relations. To interpret a text, to discover its meaning, or meanings, is to trace those relations. Reading thus becomes a process of moving between texts. Meaning becomes something which exists between a text and all the other texts to which it refers and relates, moving out from the independent text into a network of textual relations. The text becomes intertext"[31].'

'So the meaning of a text is determined by the reader as much as by the writer?'

'By the reader *instead of* the writer, according to Barthes. He claims that there is no original, authorial (authoritarian) meaning, only conscious or unconscious references to the work of other writers, which are themselves references to others, and so on, *ad infinitum*. What was it he wrote? "So the Text ... [is] woven entirely with citations, references, echoes, cultural languages (what language is not?) antecedent or contemporary, which cut across it through and through in a vast stereophony. The intertextual in which every text is held, it itself being the text-between of another text, is not to be confused with some origin of the text: to try to find the 'sources', the 'influences' of a work, is to fall in with the myth of filiation; the citations which go to make up a text are anonymous, untraceable, and yet already read: they are quotations without inverted commas"[32].'

'"Quotations without inverted commas", I like that. Or should I say, quotations without inverted commas, I like that?'

'Either will do. If I may quote again, this time from a novel by Raymond Federman:

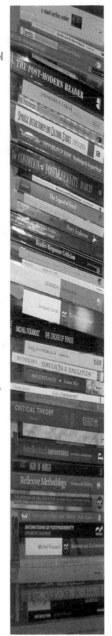

First   Person

or   ?

Third   Person

First Person is more restrictive   more subjective   more personal   harder

Third Person is more objective   more impersonal   more encompassing   easier

I could try both ways;

I was standing on the upper deck next to a girl called Mary .... No Peggy

He was standing on the upper deck next to a girl called Mary .... No Peggy

comes out the same[33].'

'So,' he said, 'first person or third person - comes out the same.'

'Or does it?' came the reply. 'If all writing is simply quotation without the inverted commas, is it really possible to write in good faith in the first person; to write "I said", when what I really mean is "S/he said"?'

'But, of course, he responded, s/he *didn't* say either, s/he merely recorded (without the inverted commas) what someone else said.'

This, of course, is a good point, and it was decided therefore to abandon the active case altogether, and to conclude simply that *it was said*. It has been claimed, then, that the individual text, along with the individual author, is a myth; a myth that possibly began with the advent of publishing as a commercial venture. Certainly, in medieval times, authorship was rarely claimed by any individual writer. The author, as Barthes might or might not have said, is a second-order fiction to authenticate the fiction of the book[34]. To provide a text with an author is to legitimise it, to own it (one might even say, to steal it). In order to prevent the text from falling into an abyss without a bottom, it must be provided with an author, and thus transformed into a work, an *oeuvre*, a book.

So where does the book begin?
Where does it end?

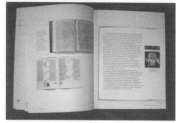

'The frontiers of a book are never clear-cut:

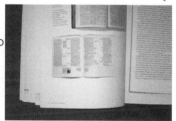

beyond the title, the first lines, and the last full stop, beyond its internal configuration and its autonomous form, it is caught up in

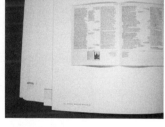

a system of references

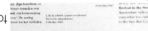

to other books, other texts, other sentences;

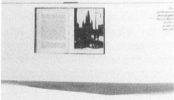

it is a node within a network'.[35]

Notes

1   Derrida, J.(1967) *Writing and Difference*, London: Routledge, 1978, p.11

2   Merleau-Ponty, cited in Derrida, ibid., p.11

3   Cixous, H. (1996) Writing Blind. In *Stigmata: Escaping Texts*, London: Routledge, 1998, p.145

4   Jabès, cited in Derrida, op. cit., p.65

5   Cixous, op. cit., p.150

6   Ibid., p.147

7   Barthes, R. (1973) *The Pleasure of the Text*, New York: Hill and Wang, 1975, pp.50-1

8   Cixous, op. cit., p.149

9   Lupton, E. & Miller, A. (1996) *Design Writing Research*, London: Phaidon Press, 1999, p.23

10 Derrida, J. Living On: Border Lines. In H. Bloom et al, *Deconstruction and Criticism*, London: Routledge and Kegan Paul, 1979, pp.83-4

11 Barthes, op. cit., p.66

12 Ibid., pp.66-7

13 All definitions are from *The New Penguin English Dictionary*, Harmondsworth, Penguin, 2001

14 Ibid., p.64

15 Barthes, R. (1975) *Roland Barthes by Roland Barthes*, Basingstoke: Macmillan, 1995, p.118

16 Ibid., p.136

17 Ibid., p.136

18 Ibid., p.136

19 Cixous, op. cit., p.140

20 Ibid., p.139

21 Barthes, op. cit., p.137

22 Cixous, H. (1990) *Three Steps on the Ladder of Writing*, New York: Columbus University Press, 1993, pp.5-6

23 Ibid., p.6

24 Jabès, E. *From the Book to the Book*, Hanover: Wesleyan University Press, 1991, p.172

25 Nietzsche, cited in Derrida, op. cit., p.29

26 Cixous, op. cit., p.64
27 Freud, cited in J. Derrida *Of Grammatology*, Baltimore: The Johns Hopkins University Press, 1974, p.p.xlvii
28 Cixous, Writing Blind, op. cit., p.149
29 Michel de Montaigne, cited in Fletcher, A. *The Art of Looking Sideways*, London: Phaidon Press, 2001, p.2
30 Barthes, R. *Image Music Text*, London: Fontana, 1977, p.146
31 Allen, G. *Intertextuality*, London: Routledge, 2000, p.1
32 Barthes, op. cit., pp.159-60
33 Federman, R. (1971) *Double or Nothing*, Normal, Illinois: Fiction Collective Two, 1998, p.139
34 Barthes, *Roland Barthes by Roland Barthes*, op. cit., p.136
35 Foucault, M. (1969) *The Archaeology of Knowledge*, London: Tavistock Publications, 1974, p.23

Afterword 3

A tissue of truths

Then perhaps it will be understood that the value of truth (and all those values associated with it) is never contested or destroyed in my writings, but only reinscribed in more powerful, larger, more stratified contexts.[1]

(p)re:text

Although we have seen that Derrida's announcement that 'there is nothing outside the text' should not be taken too literally, at times it suits him to suppose that there really *is* nothing outside the text:

> But one thing at least I can tell you now: an hour's reading beginning on any page of any one of the texts I have published over the last twenty years, should suffice for you to realise that *text*, as I use the word, is not the book. No more than writing or trace, it is not limited to the paper which you cover with your graphism. It is precisely for strategic reasons that I found it necessary to recast the concept of text by generalising it almost without limit, in any case without present or perceptible limit, without any limit that *is*. That's why there is nothing 'beyond the text'.[2]

Derrida describes a ghostly 'trace' of writing, an original, idealised *writing*, a writing that he sometimes gives the name *arche writing*, an arche writing that lies behind not only the physical process of inscribing words on paper, but also behind speech. This, of course, is why he is able to deconstruct the opposition of the binary pair Speech:writing, since each is descended from the same roots, from the same *arche*type.

> For some time now ... one says 'language' for action, movement,
> thought, reflection, consciousness, unconsciousness, experience,
> affectivity, etc. Now *we* tend to say 'writing' for all that and more: to
> designate not only the physical gestures of literal pictographic or ideo-
> graphic inscription, but also the totality of what makes it possible; and
> also, beyond the signifying face, the signified face itself. And thus we
> say 'writing' for all that gives rise to an inscription in general, whether
> it is literal or not and even if what it distributes in space is alien to the
> order of the voice: cinematography, choreography, of course, but also
> pictorial, musical, sculptural 'writing'.[3]

And also practice? Healthcare as 'writing'? What does it mean to say that
practice is a text? An *archetext*? A *book*, even? And if practice is a text,
then it is open to being deconstructed like any other text:

> That's why deconstructive readings and writings are concerned not
> only with library books, with discourses, with conceptual and
> semantic contents. They are not simply analyses of discourse.... They
> are also effective or active interventions, in particular political and
> institutional interventions that transform contexts without limiting
> themselves to theoretical or constative utterances even though they
> must produce such utterances.[4]

So, deconstruction applies not only to written texts, but to 'writing' in
its broader form, to *arche writing*. For this reason, I have been able to
deconstruct not only the texts that constitute the body of knowledge of
evidence-based practice, not only the journals that disseminate that body
of knowledge, but *evidence-based practice itself*. And I have attempted
this in a number of ways: by exposing the inconsistencies deliberately
concealed at the very heart of the dominant discourse of evidence-based
practice; by showing how the meanings of certain words are bent, distorted, in order to further the political ends of the dominant discourse; by
demonstrating how the authority of that dominant discourse is brought to
bear on competing narratives; and, on a wider stage, by arguing that the
analytic logic on which the discourse of evidence-based practice is founded is perhaps not the *only* logic.

As Lechte[5] points out, Derrida wishes to undermine the traditional
Aristotelian logic of identity, which Russell summarised as:1 Whatever is,

is; 2 Nothing can both be and not be; 3 Everything must either be or not be[6]. It is, of course, this so-called 'law of the excluded middle' that allows proponents of evidence-based practice to contrast practice based on research with practice based on 'blind conjecture, dogmatic ritual or private intuition'[7] as though there is no middle ground; as though all practice that is not research-based must, by definition, be blindly dogmatic. Does all practice have to be based *either* on research evidence *or* on conjecture and ritual? Or are supporters of evidence-based practice cynically setting up practice that is not based on research as a straw (wo)man to be knocked down by the slightest puff of wind?

I have argued elsewhere that the motivation for evidence-based practice (EBP) appears to be based on a kind of overcompensation, a 'mine is bigger than yours' attitude in which evidence (any evidence) for EBP is stacked up, piled high, in order to disguise the fact (yes, fact) that there is, in fact (yes, fact) very little evidence to support it. But of course, this strategy ultimately degenerates into what Freud typified as the logic of dreams, or 'kettle logic'. As Derrida says of this 'kettle logic':

> In his attempt to arrange everything in his favour, the defendant piles up contradictory arguments: 1. The kettle I am returning to you is brand new; 2. The holes were already in it when you lent it to me; 3. You never lent me a kettle anyway'.[8]

A more contemporary example might be described as 'Bart Simpson logic'. Thus: I didn't do it; nobody saw me do it; you can't prove it was me who did it. Or better: 'The RCT is the most appropriate design for evaluating the effectiveness of a nursing intervention'; 'Clinical expertise must prevail if the nurse decides that the patient is too frail for a specific intervention that is otherwise "best" for his condition'; 'History has shown numerous examples of [the use of clinical experience] which, on a patient by patient basis might appear to be beneficial, but when evaluated using RCTs have shown to be of doubtful value, or even harmful'[9]. To be fair, the apologists for EBP are faced with a task that contradicts their own analytic logic (nothing can both be and not be): to promote a hierarchy of evidence whilst maintaining that there is no hierarchy, that 'the key is ensuring that the right research design is used to answer the question posed'[10]. And inevitably, the fissures manifest themselves in logical inconsistencies and aporias.

This final Afterword brings together (at least) five characters. Firstly, there is Ben, a young man who has had a 'mental breakdown'. Secondly, there is Theo, a psychiatric nurse who is working with Ben and who reflects on their relationship. Thirdly, there is F, who does (at least) two things: she discusses the theory of reflective practice and she reflects on Theo's reflections *as if she was Theo*. Fourthly, there is R, who occasionally comments and theorises on F's reflections. And finally, there is the chorus, a series of voices telling a series of stories.

These characters ask (but do not answer) a number of questions, largely concerned with truth and the nature of practice. Thus, if practice is seen as a text, then to what extent and in what sense can it be said to be true? And if reflection is a story that I tell to myself, then is it nothing but a branch of fiction? And if it is...?

And finally, of course, we come to the question of endings...

Notes

1   Derrida, J. Afterword: toward an ethic of discussion. In G. Graff (ed) *Limited Inc*, Evanston, Illinois: Northwestern University Press, 1988, p.146

2   Derrida, J. But, beyond... (Open letter to Anne McClintock and Rob Nixon), *Critical Inquiry*, 1986, 13, 1, 155-70, p.167, his emphases

3   Derrida, J. (1967) *Of Grammatology*, Baltimore: The Johns Hopkins University Press, 1974, p.9

4   Derrida, But, beyond..., op. cit., p.167

5   Lechte, J. *Fifty Key Contemporary Thinkers*, London: Routledge, 1994, p.106

6   Russell, B. *The Problems of Philosophy*, Oxford: Oxford University Press, 1973, p.40

7   Blomfield, R. & Hardy, S. Evidence-based nursing practice. In S. Reynolds & L. Trinder (eds), *Evidence-Based Practice: A Critical Approach*, Oxford: Blackwell Science, 2000

8   Derrida, J. (1972) *Dissemination*, London: The Athlone Press, 1981, p.111

9   All three statements are taken from DiCenso, A., Cullum, N. & Ciliska, D. Implementing evidence-based nursing: some misconceptions, *Evidence-Based Nursing*, 1, 2, 38-40, 1998

10 Ibid., p.29

The(o's) scenario

Ben is twenty years old. I first met him in a drop-in centre for young people. I was immediately drawn to him because he was obviously a very intelligent and creative young man. Within minutes of meeting him we were discussing existentialism and modern art. His eyes would dart from side to side as he quickly weighed up the content of any conversation. I was extremely impressed with the power of his creative mind.

Over the next few times we met, it was clear to me that Ben preferred my company than to be with his peers. Ben told me that two years ago he had gone to university to study philosophy but had to give up his course because he had a mental breakdown and had been admitted to an acute mental health ward. He stayed on the ward for two weeks but discharged himself to his parents' home. Ben was now unemployed and living on his own. Ben was also angry at his parents for the way they treated him at this time. It became obvious that he was extremely unhappy, he showed me his wrists, which were freshly sutured and terribly scarred. Because I only worked at the drop-in centre one day per week I was only able to see Ben on the days I was there. Over the next few weeks, on the days I was working at the centre, Ben demanded virtually all of my time. He confided with me that he was seriously troubled with critical voices in his mind. He was bitterly angry at the way he had been treated by mental health services two years ago. Ben was insistent that mental health professionals abused him, he would not seek medical help, and he would have nothing more to do with doctors and nurses. Ben was well aware that I was a mental health nurse and I was at the centre to work with young people with problems; but it became obvious that Ben did not see me as part of the system. It also became obvious to me that Ben needed some professional help in order to keep him safe.

I eventually persuaded Ben to go along to a local GP. I went with him. His meeting with the GP was awful; she patronised him and gave him a prescription for Chlorpromazine. Ben was furious at the way he was treated by the GP and now he was also angry with me for suggesting he try the Chlorpromazine to help with his voices.

Theo's reflections

- Ben reminds me of myself when I was his age, but he is brighter than I was
- I envy his intelligence and creativity
- I wanted to befriend and help Ben
- My children have now grown up and left home
- I wanted Ben to see me as an ideal parent
- I thought about Ben many times during the week

Critical reflection: the practice of scepticism

The term 'sceptical', originating from the Greek *Skeptikos* meaning thoughtful, paying attention to and reflective, combines immersion with critical distance. Demanding that I call everyday practices into question, it requires both reflection in action and reflection on action, each of which in turn requires immersion and critical distance.

Many theories of practice (including, as I have indicated, evidence-based practice) are presented as a set of instructions to be followed, techniques for clinical effectiveness, written by experts who *know* and who expect their readers blindly to follow them. Rather like the prescription for the treatment of a disease, to be taken three times a day in order to maximise its efficacy, above all else we are urged to complete the course; that is, to follow the instructions thoroughly. In contrast, critical reflection does not diag-nose 'the disease' in terms of its underlying course or structure. In this chapter, I do not intend to prescribe critical reflection as a sort of anti-evidence based practice which claims to be a more effective technique, rather I want to foster a sceptical stance towards critical reflection. Taking a sceptical stance, the critically reflective practitioner attends to the state of conflict, allowing this to be indicative of its own treatment. As Heaton[1] frames it in his discussion of pyrrhonian scepticism, it is to 'attend to where the shoe pinches',

re:flection

The aim of deconstruction is not, of course, to replace EBP with some alternative such as reflective practice, but to point out the contradictions and aporias in each, to show that they share many of the same problems. We should therefore not be tempted to view alternatives to EBP such as reflective practice either as diametrically opposed, that is, as the second-(ary) term in a binary pair, or as itself free from the internal contradictions that beset EBP. If critical reflection is the practice of scepticism, then it demands a combination of immersion and critical distance, of subjectivity and objectivity. That is not to say, immersion *then* critical distance, subjectivity *then* objectivity, but rather (in direct contravention of Russell's second law of Aristotelian logic), subjectivity *and* objectivity.

I begin calmly, though my voice may rise as I go along[1].

to apply critique only where the practitioner feels this to be necessary.

A critical reflection, based on a sceptical practice, is thus less a technique and more an ability. It is the ability to live in uncertainty and doubt, whilst simultaneously not being paralysed by that doubt. Gordon adds 'The sceptics are inquirers but this is not the same as to seek, for in inquiry there is no end to be gained and held. Sceptical inquiry does not seek the answers'[2]. Rather it encourages us to recognise that meaning is never fixed, but is lost, found, forgotten, remembered, open to question and revision, and never closed. Seekers use their factual memory to the detriment of their perceptual memory; inquirers draw upon multiple resources to integrate experiences as they are dynamised.

In this way it is closely aligned with deconstruction, in which the impossibility of achieving consensus about what is effective practice is revealed. And like Derrida's exposition of undecidability[3], uncertainty is not a moment to be traversed or overcome; rather, it is a hyperpoliticising of the uncertainty that continues to inhabit the decision. All certainty is relative. By providing a critical reflection of the following practice narrative, what I intend to do in the subsequent discussion is to hyperpoliticise the text, making explicit some of the exclusions that live alongside the decisions.

Logic tells us that something cannot be both A and not A; experience sometimes tells us otherwise.

The problem is not that things have this ambiguous nature but that our ordinary consciousness cannot accept it ... either/or logic cannot understand the phenomenon, much less accept it and derive benefit from it.[2]

The problem lies not in reality, but in our inadequate attempts to conceptualise reality. Practice might be a text, but it's not all black and white.

This seeming logical inconsistency is a feature not only of critical reflection and EBP (which claims to support both intuition and research findings), but also of schizophrenia and, more generally, of (post)modernism[3]. Indeed, we might view both schizophrenia and (post)modernist art as critical reflection taken to its extreme, or what Louis Sass refers to as hyper-reflexivity.

*A and Not A and D suddenly Not D, no
A inverted and D passed and yet still D
but altered altering A, that is A seen
from different Ds, with the feeling of
being seen by unknown D, and also A
seen by A inside, and D seen by
SuperD.[3]*

*Oh God comma habitual self
consciousness*

Dropping in and out

*Ben is twenty years old. I first met
him in a drop-in centre for young
people. I was immediately drawn
to him because he was obviously a
very intelligent and creative young
man. Within minutes of meeting
him we were discussing existentialism and modern art. His eyes
would dart from side to side as he
quickly weighed up the content of
any conversation. I was extremely
impressed with the power of his
creative mind.*

Character, in its portrayal of human
nature and of experience, is argu-
ably the single most important
component of a reflective narrative. Lodge observes that: 'The
simplest way to introduce a
character, common in older
fiction, is to give a physical description and biographical summary[5]. But this description is
invariably highly selective, as are
the inclusion and exclusion criteria,
that is, what to keep in and what to
leave out. The criteria by which
certain aspects of the character
are portrayed and the case outlin-

For Sass, modernism and
schizophrenia both run up
against the paradox of
self-reflection as being
at once subjective *and*
objective: 'Insofar as I
focus on the world, it
will seem like *my* world;
but insofar as I focus
more directly on thoughts
or feelings, these will
seem to exist out there
and apart'[5]. The person
with schizophrenia is at
times acutely self-
conscious, we might say
hyperconscious: 'an
observer of my own mental
peculiarities, to a degree
which I think must be a
very rare exception'[6], as
one sufferer put it. But
taken just a step further,
this acute subjectivity
becomes an even more acute
objectivity, where the
self is perceived not from
within, but from without,
as detached and separate
from the observer. As Sass
observes: 'Instead of
serving as a kind of
anchoring center, the self
may be dispersed outwards,
where it fragments into

ed may even remain unknown (at some level) to the narrator. Thus, as in all case study material, it is more reflective of the character of the narrator than of the character (case) in question.

parts that float among the things of the world; even the most intimate thoughts and inclinations may appear to emanate from some external source or mysterious foreign soul, as if they were "the workings of another psyche"'[7].

LIFE-STORY

Without discarding what he'd already written he began his story afresh in a somewhat different manner. Whereas his earlier version had opened in a straight-forward documentary fashion and then degenerated or at least modulated intentionally into irrealism and dissonance he decided this time to tell his tale from start to finish in a conservative, "realistic", unself-conscious way. He being by vocation an author of novels and stories it was perhaps inevitable that one afternoon the possibility would occur to the writer of these lines that his own life might be a fiction, in which he was the leading or an accessory character.[6]

Describing the facts comes first, almost as if the facts need to be put out there by way of legitimising the narrative, painting a picture which starts at the beginning, which happens on most occasions to be the facts, interesting that although the practitioner is not describing herself explicitly, that in describing the client she is revealing some very personal characteristics of her own.

Sass notes how this dichotomy is reflected in modern art, and particularly in (post)modern literature, where it is known as *metafiction*: 'a kind of writing, a kind of discourse whose shape will be an interrogation, an endless interrogation of what it is doing while doing it, an endless denunciation of its fraudulence, of what *it* really is: an illusion (a fiction), just as life is an illusion (a fiction)'[8]. Metafiction begins at the point where inward-looking, solipsistic, self-conscious writing bifurcates: where the writer and the written suddenly divide. As Waugh observes, 'To write of "I" is to discover that the attempt to fix subjectivity in writing erases that subjectivity, constructs a new subject'[9]. Or, more accurately, a new object, a new objectivity.

Without discarding what he'd already written he began his story afresh in a somewhat different manner[7].

Beginning in the middle, past the middle, nearer three-quarters done, waiting for the end. Consider how dreadful so far: passionless, abstraction, pro, dis. And it will get worse. Can we possibly continue?[10]

The meeting place was a drop-in centre. Had Ben dropped in to see me, or had I just dropped into the centre to see Ben? What do you drop in to do in drop-in centres? The notion of a drop-in centre indicates a degree of freedom, a place that one can call in, come and go as one pleases: is this really the case? What would happen to Ben if he did not drop in? Or indeed if I did not drop in, to fulfil my commitment to work? Did Ben choose to drop in to the centre; did I choose to drop in? Or did I arrive out of a sense of obligation, of duty? Further, do I choose this duty and obligation above something else? In other words, how do I arrive at the decision to arrive at the drop-in centre, and what do I exclude in my journey?

re:Theo
What is going on here? What is F up to? This is, after all, an example from Theo's practice, Theo's reflection, The(o's) scenario, as F is quick to point out. So why does she reflect on it in the first person, why is she (para) citing Theo *as if she was he* (just as Theo wishes he was Ben)? F reflects on Theo's experience as if she was Theo, or (better), as if Theo's experience was hers. She is dropping in and out of character. She is playing a part. And as Sass reminds us, this 'uncoupling' is characteristic of the schizoid individual, in which a division is set up 'between two different selves: a hidden, "inner" self that watches or controls, usually associated with the mind, and a public, outer self that is more closely identified with bodily appearance and social role and that tends to be felt as somehow false and unreal'[11].

That is why I never ask myself 'who am I?' (qui suis-je?). I ask myself 'who are I' (qui sont-je?) - an untranslatable phrase[8].

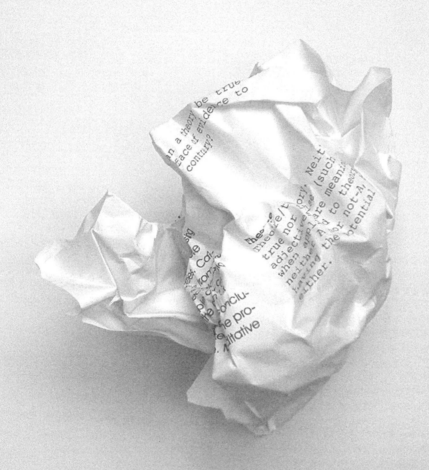

qui sont-je?
who are I?

qui songe?
who muses/
     dreams/
     reflects?

I reflect that I 'was drawn to' Ben because of his intelligence and creativity and that 'within minutes we were discussing existentialism and modern art' and indeed I was 'extremely impressed with the power' of Ben's creative mind. What aspects of the character and the case collide here? I also acknowledge that I want to befriend Ben. As I read my words now, I feel like I am engaged in a confessional practice. This is based on the belief that professional boundaries are rigid and that 'befriending' patients is wrong; that to have a close relationship with a patient is not only unprofessional, but also unhealthy, maybe even pathological.

He had emerged from infancy with his "own self" on the one hand, and "what his mother wanted him to be", his "personality", on the other; he had started from there and made it his aim and ideal to make the split between his own self (which only he knew) and what other people could see of him, as complete as possible[19].

An inner, authentic self (S) and an outer, public, 'false' self; an imaginary self (S^i). Or would the evidence-based practitioners say: an inner, unknown, unknowable self, an imaginary self (S^i); and an outer, public, true self (S).

a new objectivity ...   I am becoming confused ...

But the reader! Even if his author were his only reader as was he himself of his work-in-progress as of the sentence in progress and his protagonist of his, et cetera, his character as reader was not the same as his character as author, a fact which might be turned to account. What suspense[9].

Perhaps the client here is not the client but the practitioner! Here, Theo is also making public issues of his personal troubles in relation to Ben, which need to be treated with care. What is this culture about? Frank argues that this making personal troubles public issues is the foundation of politics. Thus, reflective practice could be considered a political concern.

Over the next few times we met, it was clear to me that Ben preferred my company than to be with his peers.

Emerson[10] notes that 'A friend is a person with whom I may be sin-

F^i has split from F. The F^i who writes (from) the experience of Theo is not the true, authentic F, not the F that only she knows. F^i is writing not from her experience, but from her imagination. Not a proper reflection, then. Only a fiction (a f^iction), a made-up story, a tale narrated by (in) the first person (I) to the second person (you) about the third person (Theo). A fictional I; not the practitioner, but someone pretending to be the practitioner. A false I. An impossible I. An I^i. As Russell (again appealing to Aristotelian logic) tells us: 'There are no unreal individuals, so that the null-class is the class containing no members, not the class containing as members, all unreal individuals'[13]. Not $\{I^i\}$ but $\{\quad\}$; that is, $\{\quad\}^i$.

But is 'real' reflection any different, any better, any less fictional? Can I really be sure, when I reflect, that the I who narrates the reflective account is the same I who had the experience that is

cere. Before him I may think aloud'. Perhaps it is safer to think aloud with my patients than it is to reflect aloud with my peers and colleagues. After all, to think aloud is to listen to myself talking to myself; something my patients might understand better than my colleagues. For Emerson, then, sincerity permits thinking aloud; it has no secrets. Sincere practice therefore involves the articulation of process; of the thinking, the rationale, that supports and underpins practice. To be sincere in practice, as in friendship, entails putting your cards on the table, showing your hand, revealing the evidence on which your practice is based. Similarly, Adam Phillips' view of therapeutic practice is that it is 'closer to friendship than to a doctor-patient relationship'[11]. Gordon[12], linking this to the concept of professional boundaries, writes of what constitutes evidence of a good friendship. Two of the attributes he describes are a distance that does not pretend to be objective and a faith in the other. I shall explore these attributes further, relating them to the notion of taking the other seriously, and of dependence. But this also links to authenticity, which is created in the process of storytelling. Authenticity is dialogical, it is not a pre-condition of the telling. Dialogic relationships are both the topic of the story, its content and also the goal of telling the story, its process[13]. Authenticity is interpersonal.

being reflected on? That the I who reflects on action is the I who was involved in the action? That the I who tells the story is the I about whom the story is told? Or, is the assumed equivalence between the I who writes and the I who is the subject of the writing merely a literary device, a rhetorical strategy, a story told in the first person? So who, then, is this character, this I[i] that/who writes?

a new objectivity

I do not say 'I am going to describe myself', but 'I am writing a text and I call it R.B.' ... I myself am my own symbol. I am the story which happens to me: freewheeling in language, I have nothing to compare myself to; and in this movement, the pronoun of the imaginary 'I' is im-pertinent; the symbolic becomes literally immediate: essential danger for the life of the subject: to write onself may seem a pretentious idea; but it is also a simple idea: simple as the idea of suicide.[14]

AUTOBIOGRAPHY
You who listen give me life in a manner
of speaking. I won't hold you res-
ponsible. My first words weren't my
first words. I wish I'd begun differently.
Among other things I haven't a proper
name...[14]

The writer becomes the
text; the text becomes the
writer. As John Barth says
of one of his short
stories: 'The title "Autobiography" means "self-
composition": the antece-
dent of the first-person
pronoun is not I, but the
story, speaking of itself.
I am its father; its
mother is the recording
machine'[15]. The I^i is the
story itself.

I must compose myself. Look, I'm
writing[15].

No, listen, I'm nothing
but talk; I won't last
long.[16]

authenticity is   dialogical

We have both 'fallen' for each
other, Ben declares his preference
for me...

And what of F? In
deconstructing Theo's
reflections, is she not in
danger of becoming too
close; of wanting to
become Theo's friend; of
wanting to become Theo? In
putting herself in Theo's
shoes, is she perhaps
beginning to feel the
pinch?

Ben told me that two years ago he
had gone to university to study
philosophy but had to give up his
course because he had a mental
breakdown and had been admit-
ted to an acute mental health
ward. He stayed on the ward for
two weeks but discharged himself
to his parents' home. Ben was now
unemployed and living on his own.
Ben was also angry at his parents
for the way they treated him at this
time.

The book is a dialogue or a dialectic.
At least it should be[17]

I wish I'd begun differ-
ently.

In confessing that he discharged himself, Ben indicates how he manages to assert his choice, his individuality and his freedom. Or does he? For in discharging himself, he risks the trappings of labelling and of being stereotyped as 'difficult' and 'unwell'. I often ponder what would happen if I discharged myself from my 'role' and became the creative artistic intelligent young man that I so admired (and remembered). When, in passing, I had mused on leaving the profession, my friends and colleagues had responded with cries of 'you must be mad' and 'but you have worked so hard to be who/where you are now'.

I wish I'd begun differently.

Dependence

It became obvious that he was extremely unhappy, he showed me his wrists, which were freshly sutured and terribly scarred. Because I only worked at the drop-in centre one day per week I was only able to see Ben on the days I was there. Over the next few weeks, on the days I was working at the centre, Ben demanded virtually all of my time.

Re:search

F^i wishes to stand in Theo's shoes, just as Theo wishes to stand in Ben's shoes. Inevitably, they will pinch a little. One shoe might pinch more than the other. Perhaps they are not even a pair (Derrida would certainly question this).

Yes, let us suppose for example two (laced) right shoes or two left shoes. They no longer form a pair, but the whole thing squints or limps, I don't know, in strange, worrying, perhaps threatening and slightly diabolical fashion. I sometimes have this impression with some of van Gogh's shoes and I wonder whether Schapiro and Heidegger aren't hastening to make them into a pair in order to reassure themselves. Prior to all reflection you reassure yourself with the pair[18].

Prior to all reflection, you reassure yourself with the pair... A binary pair? But I digress. To stand in someone else's shoes: hermeneutics. That is, a research method by which the researcher imagines herself *standing* in the shoes of the writer, better to under*stand* some ancient text. Or, in this case, a reflective method by which F imagines herself in Theo's shoes, by which she writes *as if she was* Theo, better to understand his experience. That is, to act as a go-between, a messenger,

Sutherland[16] observes that a characteristic of patients with mental health problems is that they are apt to become dependant on those caring for them. In particular, he suggests that the patient relies upon the carer for hope of recovery and is extremely sensitive to promises which, he argues along with other writers, are often made glibly, and are easily broken, thereby constituting a failure in the therapeutic relationship, although not one that that is necessarily overt or realised. As Sutherland notes: 'A broken promise not only causes pain but is also bad therapy'[17]. Handling patients' dependence can be a difficult balance for the practitioner. However, an added weight is that of managing her own dependence.

It is, for example, difficult for me to admit that I preferred the company of Ben to that of my peers and colleagues, and that I too looked forward to seeing him during my days at the centre. I found myself thinking about him on my days off, particularly as I browsed the bookshops in my search for existentialist philosophy.

between the writer of the text, the practitioner of the therapy, and you, the reader. After Hermes, perhaps, the messenger of the gods. (Not shoes, then, but winged sandals). A reflective/subjective approach to research. The opening of the text to the outside world, to the influence of the researcher. Another contradiction, though: hermetic, surely from the same root, meaning an airtight seal, the *exclusion* of the outside world. Hermetic:hermeneutic; Objective:subjective; Fact:fiction. Whence should we orientate our reflection, our research?

Is all reflection better described as hermeneutic phenomenology? When I reflect on action am I merely putting my 'reflective self' in the shoes of my 'practising self' and hoping that they don't pinch too much? Is *all* reflective practice nothing but a fiction? In other words, does F's reflection on Theo's practice have any more or less validity than Theo's reflection on his own practice? That is, is it any less true?

*In my search for
existentialist
philosophy...*

Being taken seriously ... or not

He confided with me that he was seriously troubled with critical voices in his mind. He was bitterly angry at the way he had been treated by mental health services two years ago. Ben was insistent that mental health professionals abused him, he would not seek medical help, and he would have nothing more to do with doctors and nurses. Ben was well aware that I was a mental health nurse and I was at the centre to work with young people with problems; but it became obvious that Ben did not see me as part of the system. It also became obvious to me that Ben needed some professional help in order to keep him safe.

Much has been written about the treatment, or rather maltreatment, of people with mental health problems,, particularly in the 1960s when novels such as *One Flew Over the Cuckoo's Nest* appeared and authors such as Laing were cultivating their exaggerated antipsychiatric stance. Simultaneously, studies of the experience of the pseudo patient were also being reported[18, 19]. The reports of the 'false' patients (the characters) were being taken more seriously than the reports of the 'real' patients (the cases), for whom the experience of being institutionalised did not lead to the development of an academic voice. Even Sutherland (himself a 'real' case) writes 'Most of the remarks made by the patients on my wards were quite sensible, with

It is tempting to think that fiction is, by definition, false; that is, not true. This binary pair Fact:fiction is both dangerous and seductive, since it makes an appeal to the binary pair Truth:falsity. Thus, if facts are true, then fiction must be false. But, as Russell would surely have pointed out, to say that facts are true does not imply that the term 'fact' is logically equivalent to the term 'true', just as we can say that two plus two equals four but not that two plus to is equivalent to four. Thus, whereas all facts are (by definition) true, not all truth is fact. There are, perhaps, other kinds of truth. Similarly, we might say that 2+2 is always 4, but that 4 is not always 2+2; it can also be 1+3, for example.

So, if there is no logical equivalence between fact and truth, there is likewise no necessary logical equivalence between fiction and falsity. Just because F's reflection on Theo's experience is (we might say) fictional does not mean that it is a false or untrue account. And perhaps we can say the same of the insights (reflections?) achieved through deconstruction.

the exception of those of a florid
schizophrenic: they, therefore,
deserved to be taken seriously'[20].
What of the remarks made by the
florid schizophrenic?

So what of the remarks
made by the florid schizophrenic? Is there any
sense in which they can be
said to be true? And what
of the 'true' patient?
*(That's right, true, not
false.)* Perhaps the problems reported in identifying the real patients from
the false are precisely
that true patients have
about them an air of falsity, 'giving the impres-
sion that they are only
role-playing'[19]. As Laing
said of his patient David,
'his ideal was, *never to
give himself away to
others*'[20].

It is very damaging to be ignored
or dismissed to those of us who are
relatively 'sane'. It is even worse to
have one's memory of events challenged by professionals. What is the
impact on the self when one's
memory of significant events is
repeatedly overruled; when others
convince you that an emotionally
significant event did not happen or
happened in a radically different
manner than you remember it? This
can lead to perpetuation of the
social isolation, persecution and
excruciating self-doubt frequently
associated with psychiatric disorders. The patient becomes the
social construct of a mentally
disordered individual.

In my search for existen-
tialist philosophy; the
philosophy of authenticity

   Being ignored and not taken
seriously (especially by those experts in supposed authority upon
whom we depend) can be the
most demoralising experience of
all[21]. Sutherland again reports, concerning his own experience as a

*The truth of the book is decidable. This
false dialogue constituted by the book
is not necessarily a dialogue that is
false.[21]*

patient being treated for a severe depressive episode: 'I knew exactly what tablets I was supposed to receive: when, as quite frequently happened, I was given the wrong ones, I would complain'. He goes on to say that 'The error was not put right: instead, I pictured the nurse going to the day book and writing, 'patient paranoid about his tab-lets'[22].

How often are practitioners taken seriously, particularly when they step outside of the system? As other chapters in this book demon-strate, often the practitioner's voice is ignored or dismissed, not least in the application of the 'hierarchy of evidence' model. Indeed how many practitioners have question-ed the actions of another member of staff, and have been ignored, only to go away shamefaced and paranoid? Some of my own reflect-ive questioning could be interpret-ed, not as reflection on action, but as latent paranoia, triggered not only by the visit to the GP, but by working within a system that views the critical voice as one to be ig-nored. Not to mention the inclusion of my own (inner) critical voices; perhaps I am the one that needed the Chlorpromazine.

Are Ben's comments about being abused by mental health professionals not to be taken seri-ously (he is after all mentally ill)? Or perhaps you, the reader, will take my comments more seriously than Ben's (after all I am the profession-al).

Since the deconstructionist (which is to say, isn't it, the skeptic-relativist-nihilist!) is supposed not to believe in truth, stability, or the unity of meaning, in intention or 'meaning-to-say', how can he demand of us that we read him with pertinence, precision, rigor? How can he demand that his own text be interpreted correctly? How can he accuse anyone else of having misunderstood, simplified, deformed it, etc? In other words, how can he discuss, and discuss the reading of what he writes? The answer is simple enough: this definition of the deconstructionist is false (that's right: false, not true) and feeble; it supposes a bad (that's right: bad, not good) and feeble reading of numerous texts, first of all mine, which therefore must finally be read or reread. Then perhaps it will be understood that the value of truth (and all those values associated with it) is never contested or destroyed in my writings, but only reinscribed in more powerful, larger, more stratified contexts[22].

Is Derrida finally showing his true colours? Has he at last found a comfort-able pair (yes, pair) of shoes?

The politics of practice: reflection as 'scientific method'

Reflective writing provides excellent journalism but is seemingly not scientific, as Roberts comments (speaking of Sutherland's work) 'I think that Professor Sutherland has bravely written subjectively and in doing so abdicated his professorship'[23]. I understand this as being true to oneself, which requires attention to that which is beyond oneself; it requires values to the things that matter to oneself and to moral ideals. Is there something wrong with the making and recording of observations (subjectively) in clinical practice; the method of critical reflection?

Heidegger distinguishes between 'calculative thinking' and 'meditative thinking'. Evidence-based practice, according to this scheme, is typified by calculative thinking or 'thinking-as-a-means-to-an-end', where the end is external to the process. Thus, 'calculative thinking computes. It computes ever new, ever more promising and at the same time more economical possibilities. Calculative thinking races from one prospect to the next. Calculative thinking never stops, never collects itself'[24]. In contrast, reflection could be seen as an example of meditative thinking, the aim of which is not to reach any conclu-

The value of the book (true/false) is not intrinsic to it. A span of writing is worth nothing in itself; it is neither good nor bad, neither true nor false.[23]

Heidegger recalls a similar story concerning Galileo. When he found that the measuring instruments of the day were not sensitive enough to provide evidence for his theory of gravity, '... *against* the evidence of experience, Galileo upheld his proposition.... By reason of this experiment the opposition towards Galileo increased to such an extent that he had to give up his professorship and leave Pisa'[24]. Resisting the dominant paradigm of EBP can be costly.

Or can a theory be true in the face of evidence to the contrary?

Theo:re
Theo:re/theory. Neither true nor false (such adjectives are meaningless when applied to theory), neither A nor not-A, but having the potential for either.

sions, but simply to keep the process of thinking alive. Meditative
thinking is therefore an end in itself,
and for Heidegger, it is only when
we are engaged in meditative
thinking that we are truly human;
that is, truly being a friend; truly
being a therapist.

*To me theories are safe but temporary
stepping stones across the dangerous
waters of life, the unknown. But it is the
unknown, not theories or principles,
that are the source of the new.... To
make theory the master of practice is
surely a form of repression.*[25]

A form of repression...

The philosophy of
authenticity...

Powerlessness

The consequence of many of the
above behaviours is powerlessness.
Powerlessness for the patient, who
becomes a victim not of mental
illness *per se*, but of the *treatment*
of her mental illness. One might
assume that if the patient is the
victim in the story, then the practitioner must be the agent. Power
has been a theme throughout
many of the chapters in this volume. Stripped of personal belong-
ings and identities, they (decide to)
enter into the world of professional
practice to be confronted with....

A theory does not have a
truth-value; it is neither
true nor not-true. Once
its truth status is established, it is either ac-
cepted or rejected as
something *other than* a
theory; as a law, perhaps.

(You should be thinking about ending it
now)

There is but one truly
serious philosophical
problem...

When looked at from the patient's point of view, withholding of information, being ignored, not being supported through the terror of dependent relationships, all are linked to power and control.

Ben decides to die.

However, all of these things can be said to be true for the practitioner, who is subject to similar abusive behaviours. Thus, instead of practice being a potential space where we are invited to come out of ourselves, where there might be hospitality, a place to dwell, to recollect and reflect, It becomes a place for fostering dependence. Facing oppression, battling for (or being overloaded by) information, stripped of personal beliefs and values in the guise of maintaining professional practice, devoid of creativity, practitioners struggle to have their own practical wisdom taken seriously.

I eventually persuaded Ben to go along to a local GP. I went with him. His meeting with the GP was awful; she patronised him and gave him a prescription for Chlorpromazine. Ben was furious at the way he was treated by the GP and now he was also angry with me for suggesting he try the Chlorpromazine to help with his voices.

```
... the problem of how to
continue in an absurd
world.
```

(I do think that you should be drawing to a conclusion)

There is but one truly serious philosophical problem and that is suicide.[26]

```
The problem of suicide is,
without doubt, an existen-
tial problem, a problem of
existence. For the exist-
entialists, the only truth
in an absurd world is to
be true to yourself, that
is, to be authentic.
```

I am taking the liberty at this point of calling the existential attitude philosophical suicide.[27]

(You really ought to be tying up the loose ends at this point)

```
To be authentic is to act
in good faith, to recog-
nise that there are no
predetermined answers to
the problems of life; that
life is a series of unique
and unforeseeable choices.
```

The end begins, this is a citation. Maybe a citation[28]

What choice does Ben have here? If he takes the medication he has 'given in', and if he doesn't take the medication, his label of being mentally ill is confirmed.

The relationship between powerlessness and paranoia is intimate; hence the experience of disempowerment perpetuates the paranoia.

Autonomous practice is self-reflective practice, but not based on self-centred individualism; such autonomous reflective practice is inextricably linked to the wider society which is fully realised in a collective reflexive democracy. Democracy can only be lived if there are democratic individuals. This is in contrast with heteronomy, in which the values, norms and principles of tradition are imposed upon individuals in an unquestioning and un-reflective way. How does reflective practice foster this? For reflective practice itself runs the risk of becoming another tradition imposed through the media of mandatory clinical supervision.

Loss of agency ... both the client and the practitioner, anger and keeping Ben out of services, what is my fear here? Autonomous practice is also practice based on scepticism.

The existentialist starts from the premise, as Sartre puts it, that existence precedes essence. We do not come into existence with a predetermined purpose in life; first we exist, and only then do we create our essence, our purpose in life.

But if existence precedes essence, then there is no essential human nature; we are determined by our choices and by nothing else. Social or psychological research cannot help us in these choices; there is no body of evidence on which to base our unique existential choices; we must choose for ourselves, without outside help. To base our choices on some imaginary 'laws' of human nature is to act in bad faith; *mauvaise foi*. The only bad choice is to choose to believe that we have no choice.

(End it! NOW!)

re:turning
To conclude? I don't think so. A conclusion suggests an end, a goal that has been achieved through some well-conceived strategy. But as Derrida observed at the end of the 'defence' of his PhD thesis:

What tradition have I fallen into in my reflection on Theo's work? Critical feminist theories, the rebellious voice of the oppressed, the skeptic? Is this the role I am supposed to take, or am I inquiring, as discussed earlier, exploring alternative stances?

You are free, therefore choose - that is to say, invent.[25]

Weber's great question is *what stand shall I take?* Tolstoy poses the dilemma: science is meaningless because it gives no answer to our question, the only question important to us, the question of what shall we do and how shall we live. Theo's questions to himself are all taking him back to this point. What solutions does he find through reflections, *if indeed solutions are the answer*. The local and the contingent that recount past attempted solutions through reflective practice are expressed as stories, these are the solutions to how we should live and are part of our ongoing attempts to seek present ways of living[26].

The blank of our lives. It's about over. Let the dénouement be soon and unexpected, painless if possible, quick at least, above all soon. Not now! How in the world will it ever[27]

You have heard too much talk of strategies. Strategy is a word that I have perhaps abused in the past, especially as it has been always only to specify in the end, in an apparently self-contradictory manner and at the risk of cutting the ground from under my own feet - something I almost never fail to do - that this strategy is a strategy without any finality; for this is what I hold and what in turn holds me in its grip, the aleatory strategy of someone who admits that he does not know where he is going. This, then, is not after all an undertaking of war or a discourse of belligerence. I should like it to be also like a headlong flight straight towards the end, a joyous self-contradiction, a disarmed desire, that is to say something very old and very cunning, but which also has just been born and which delights in being without defence[29].

(Well, if not a conclusion, then what about a summary? F appears to be attempting one)

How can a book conclude when it does not know where it is going on its 'headlong flight straight towards the end'? A joyous self-contradiction. But isn't that what Derrida does best? And as he adds elsewhere, 'A book neither begins nor ends: at most
continued on p.3

Notes

1　Heaton, J. M. Pyrrhonian scepticism: a therapeutic phenomenology. *Journal of the British Society for Phenomenology,* 28, *1997*

2　Gordon, P. *Face to Face. Therapy as Ethics,* London: Constable, 1999, p.158

3　Derrida, J. Remarks on Deconstruction and Pragmatism. In C. Mouffe (ed) *Deconstruction and Pragmatism,* London: Routledge, 1996, Ch 7

4　Cixous, H. *Déluge,* Paris: Des Femmes, 1992, p.226

5　Lodge, D. *The Art of Fiction,* London: Penguin, 1992, p.67

6　Barth, J. *Lost in the Funhouse,* New York: Anchor Books, 1988, p.116

7　Ibid., p.116

8　Cixous, H. Preface. In S. Sellers (ed) *The Hélèn Cixous Reader,* London: Routledge, 1994, p.xvii

9　Barth, op. cit., p.123

10　Emerson, R.W. (1841) *Friendship,* New York: Souvenir Press, 1988

11　Phillips, A. Comment. *The Guardian,* 14th March 1998

12　Gordon, op. cit.

13　Frank, A. Why study people's stories? The dialogical ethics of narrative analysis, *International Journal of Qualitative Methods,* 1, (1), 6, Winter 2002

14　Barth, op. cit., p.35

15　Ibid., p.36

16　Sutherland, S. What goes wrong in the care and treatment of the mentally ill. In W. Dryden and C. Feltham (eds) *Psycho-*

Notes

1　Barth, J. *Lost in the Funhouse,* New York: Anchor Books, 1988, p.110

2　Weil, A. *The Natural Mind,* Harmondsworth: Penguin, 1975, pp.146-7

3　Sass, L. *Madness and Modernism,* Cambridge Mass: Harvard University Press, 1992

4　Barth, op. cit., p.113

5　Sass, op. cit., p.338

6　Cited by Sass, op. cit., p.227

7　Ibid., p.324. Sass is quoting Bleueler

8　Federman, R. Surfiction - four propositions in the form of an introduction. In R. Federman (ed) *Surfiction: Fiction Now and Tomorrow,* Chicago: Swallow Press, 1975, p.11

9　Waugh, P. *Metafiction: The Theory and Practice of Self-Conscious Fiction,* London: Routledge, 1984, p.135

10　Barth, op. cit., p.105

11　Sass, op. cit., p.97

12　Laing, R. *The Divided Self,* Harmondsworth: Penguin, 1965, p.71

13　Russell, B. On denoting, *Mind,* 14, 1905

14　Barthes, R. *Roland Barthes by Roland Barthes,* London: Macmillan, 1977, p.56

15　Barth, op. cit., p.203

16　Ibid., p.36

17　Derrida, J. *Acts of Literature,* New York: Routledge, 1992, p.131

therapy and its discontents, Open University Press: Buckingham, 1992, Ch 7

17 Ibid., p.174

18 Deane, W.N. Reactions of a non-patient to a stay on a mental hospital ward. *Psychiatry*, 1961, 24, 61-68

19 Goldman, A.R. On posing as mental patients: reminiscences and recommendations. *Professional Psychology*, 1970, 1 427-434

20 Sutherland, op. cit., p.177

21 Gotkin, J. and Gotkin, P. *Too much anger, Too many tears*, London: Jonathan Cape, 1977

22 Sutherland, op. cit., p.177

23 Roberts, J. Response to Stuart Sutherland. In W. Dryden and C. Feltham (eds) *Psychotherapy and its Discontents*, Open University Press: Buckingham, 1992, p.190

24 Heidegger, M. *Discourse on Thinking*, New York: Harper & Row, 1966, p.46

25 Sartre, J.-P. *Existentialism and Humanism*, London: Eyre Methuen, 1973, p.38

26 Frank, op. cit.

27 Barth, J. (1963) Title. In J. Barth *Lost in the Funhouse*, New York: Anchor Books, 1988, p.113

18 Derrida, J. (1978) Restitutions of the truth in pointing. In P. Kamuf (ed) *A Derrida Reader*, Hemel Hempstead: Harvester Wheatsheaf, 1991, pp.287-8

19 Sass, op. cit., p.77

20 Laing, op. cit., p.71

21 Derrida, *Acts of Literature*, op. cit., p.132

22 Derrida, D. *Limited Inc*, Evanston: Northwestern University Press, 1988, p.146

23 Derrida, *Acts of Literature*, op. cit., p.133

24 Heidegger, M. *Basic Writings*, London: Routledge, 1993, p.290

25 Jones, J.C. *Designing Designing*, London: Architecture Design and Technology Press, 1991, p.7

26 Camus, A. *The Myth of Sisyphus*, Harmondsworth: Penguin, 1975, p.11

27 Ibid., p.43

28 Derrida, *Acts of Literature*, op. cit., p.231

29 Derrida, J. The time of a thesis: punctuations. In A. Montefiore (ed) *Philosophy in France Today*, Cambridge: Cambridge University Press, p.50

Author, have you ever written the book you wanted to write?
Have I ever wanted to write a book and believed I was writing it?
I've tried. In the end a book is left. And I adopt it.

Helen Cixous 1990

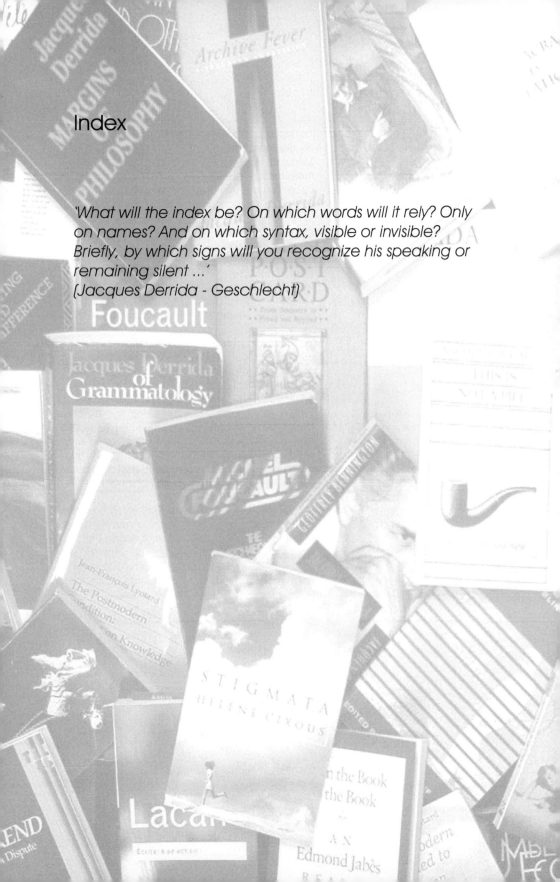

Index

'What will the index be? On which words will it rely? Only on which words will it rely? Only on names? And on which syntax, visible or invisible? Briefly, by which signs will you recognize his speaking or remaining silent ...'
(Jacques Derrida - Geschlecht)

At last, we come to the index

Beyond the text, at the edge of the book

Caught between the text and the back cover

Deconstruction, 1-215
Derrida, 1-215

Entries should be arranged systematic-ally, in alphabetical order, word by word, using subheads and cross references where necessary
Evidence-based practice, 1-215

Finger, index [Latin *indic-*, *index* fore-finger, informer, guide, from indicare]. In printing, a character in the form of a point-ing hand that directs a reader to a note, cross-reference, etc.

G ☞ *see* H

However, we have seen the difficulties involved in accurate pointing; in pointing at/to the truth. It is not, as we have seen, that there is no truth, but rather that I have no guarantee that you will follow the line of my pointing finger.
☞ *see also* Postman

of Truth

Index, 219
It is important to iden-tify the most relevant items and to discrimi-nate, excluding only passing mentions of a subject or topic.

Just who decides what are the most relevant items and what should be excluded? And who *should* decide? The writer? The reader?

Knowledge manage-ment has become one of the most important skills in a world over-flowing with evidence. Why read the book when you need only read the index in order to extricate the most relevant items?

List ☞ *see* Index
an alphabetical list of names, topics, etc mentioned in a printed work indicating the page number or num-bers where the items appear
Location
The index should provide the user with an efficient means of locating information; or

Maybe

Not

Or maybe

Postman of Truth, The
There is always the possibility that the letter does not arrive; that it is delivered to the wrong address... 'The postman of truth, the ...

... Question of the delivery of truth in psychoanalysis'

Really, then, the index is nothing more than a

Systematic guide or list to aid reference

The best person to compile an index is the author, who has a good knowledge of the subject and an appreciation of the ideas and presenta-tion of the material

Ultimately, then, if the reader has replaced the writer as the 'author' of the text, then shouldn't you be the one to complete this index?

V

We're waiting...

X

Y

Zzzz